Mometrix
TEST PREPARATION

CRNFA®

Exam Secrets Study Guide

I0878039

Dear Future Exam Success Story

First of all, **THANK YOU** for purchasing Mometrix study materials!

Second, congratulations! You are one of the few determined test-takers who are committed to doing whatever it takes to excel on your exam. **You have come to the right place.** We developed these study materials with one goal in mind: to deliver you the information you need in a format that's concise and easy to use.

In addition to optimizing your guide for the content of the test, we've outlined our recommended steps for breaking down the preparation process into small, attainable goals so you can make sure you stay on track.

We've also analyzed the entire test-taking process, identifying the most common pitfalls and showing how you can overcome them and be ready for any curveball the test throws you.

Standardized testing is one of the biggest obstacles on your road to success, which only increases the importance of doing well in the high-pressure, high-stakes environment of test day. Your results on this test could have a significant impact on your future, and this guide provides the information and practical advice to help you achieve your full potential on test day.

Your success is our success

We would love to hear from you! If you would like to share the story of your exam success or if you have any questions or comments in regard to our products, please contact us at **800-673-8175** or **support@mometrix.com**.

Thanks again for your business and we wish you continued success!

Sincerely,
The Mometrix Test Preparation Team

Written and edited by the Mometrix Exam Secrets Test Prep Team
Printed in the United States of America

TABLE OF CONTENTS

Introduction

Thank you for purchasing this resource! You have made the choice to prepare yourself for a test that could have a huge impact on your future, and this guide is designed to help you be fully ready for test day. Obviously, it's important to have a solid understanding of the test material, but you also need to be prepared for the unique environment and stressors of the test, so that you can perform to the best of your abilities.

For this purpose, the first section that appears in this guide is the **Secret Keys**. We've devoted countless hours to meticulously researching what works and what doesn't, and we've boiled down our findings to the five most impactful steps you can take to improve your performance on the test. We start at the beginning with study planning and move through the preparation process, all the way to the testing strategies that will help you get the most out of what you know when you're finally sitting in front of the test.

We recommend that you start preparing for your test as far in advance as possible. However, if you've bought this guide as a last-minute study resource and only have a few days before your test, we recommend that you skip over the first two Secret Keys since they address a long-term study plan.

If you struggle with **test anxiety**, we strongly encourage you to check out our recommendations for how you can overcome it. Test anxiety is a formidable foe, but it can be beaten, and we want to make sure you have the tools you need to defeat it.

Secret Key 1: Plan Big, Study Small

There's a lot riding on your performance. If you want to ace this test, you're going to need to keep your skills sharp and the material fresh in your mind. You need a plan that lets you review everything you need to know while still fitting in your schedule. We'll break this strategy down into three categories.

Information Organization

Start with the information you already have: the official test outline. From this, you can make a complete list of all the concepts you need to cover before the test. Organize these concepts into groups that can be studied together, and create a list of any related vocabulary you need to learn so you can brush up on any difficult terms. You'll want to keep this vocabulary list handy once you actually start studying since you may need to add to it along the way.

Time Management

Once you have your set of study concepts, decide how to spread them out over the time you have left before the test. Break your study plan into small, clear goals so you have a manageable task for each day and know exactly what you're doing. Then just focus on one small step at a time. When you manage your time this way, you don't need to spend hours at a time studying. Studying a small block of content for a short period each day helps you retain information better and avoid stressing over how much you have left to do. You can relax knowing that you have a plan to cover everything in time. In order for this strategy to be effective though, you have to start studying early and stick to your schedule. Avoid the exhaustion and futility that comes from last-minute cramming!

Study Environment

The environment you study in has a big impact on your learning. Studying in a coffee shop, while probably more enjoyable, is not likely to be as fruitful as studying in a quiet room. It's important to keep distractions to a minimum. You're only planning to study for a short block of time, so make the most of it. Don't pause to check your phone or get up to find a snack. It's also important to **avoid multitasking**. Research has consistently shown that multitasking will make your studying dramatically less effective. Your study area should also be comfortable and well-lit so you don't have the distraction of straining your eyes or sitting on an uncomfortable chair.

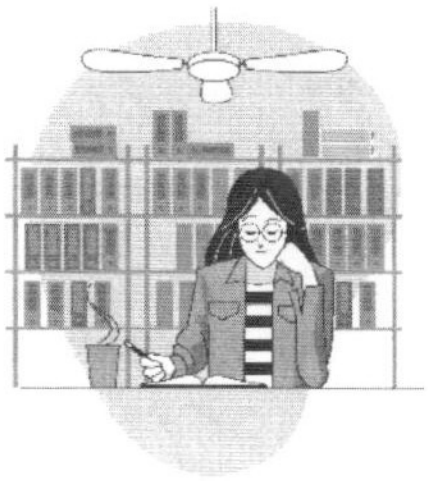

The time of day you study is also important. You want to be rested and alert. Don't wait until just before bedtime. Study when you'll be most likely to comprehend and remember. Even better, if you know what time of day your test will be, set that time aside for study. That way your brain will be used to working on that subject at that specific time and you'll have a better chance of recalling information.

Finally, it can be helpful to team up with others who are studying for the same test. Your actual studying should be done in as isolated an environment as possible, but the work of organizing the information and setting up the study plan can be divided up. In between study sessions, you can discuss with your teammates the concepts that you're all studying and quiz each other on the details. Just be sure that your teammates are as serious about the test as you are. If you find that your study time is being replaced with social time, you might need to find a new team.

Secret Key 2: Make Your Studying Count

You're devoting a lot of time and effort to preparing for this test, so you want to be absolutely certain it will pay off. This means doing more than just reading the content and hoping you can remember it on test day. It's important to make every minute of study count. There are two main areas you can focus on to make your studying count.

Retention

It doesn't matter how much time you study if you can't remember the material. You need to make sure you are retaining the concepts. To check your retention of the information you're learning, try recalling it at later times with minimal prompting. Try carrying around flashcards and glance at one or two from time to time or ask a friend who's also studying for the test to quiz you.

To enhance your retention, look for ways to put the information into practice so that you can apply it rather than simply recalling it. If you're using the information in practical ways, it will be much easier to remember. Similarly, it helps to solidify a concept in your mind if you're not only reading it to yourself but also explaining it to someone else. Ask a friend to let you teach them about a concept you're a little shaky on (or speak aloud to an imaginary audience if necessary). As you try to summarize, define, give examples, and answer your friend's questions, you'll understand the concepts better and they will stay with you longer. Finally, step back for a big picture view and ask yourself how each piece of information fits with the whole subject. When you link the different concepts together and see them working together as a whole, it's easier to remember the individual components.

Finally, practice showing your work on any multi-step problems, even if you're just studying. Writing out each step you take to solve a problem will help solidify the process in your mind, and you'll be more likely to remember it during the test.

Modality

Modality simply refers to the means or method by which you study. Choosing a study modality that fits your own individual learning style is crucial. No two people learn best in exactly the same way, so it's important to know your strengths and use them to your advantage.

For example, if you learn best by visualization, focus on visualizing a concept in your mind and draw an image or a diagram. Try color-coding your notes, illustrating them, or creating symbols that will trigger your mind to recall a learned concept. If you learn best by hearing or discussing information, find a study partner who learns the same way or read aloud to yourself. Think about how to put the information in your own words. Imagine that you are giving a lecture on the topic and record yourself so you can listen to it later.

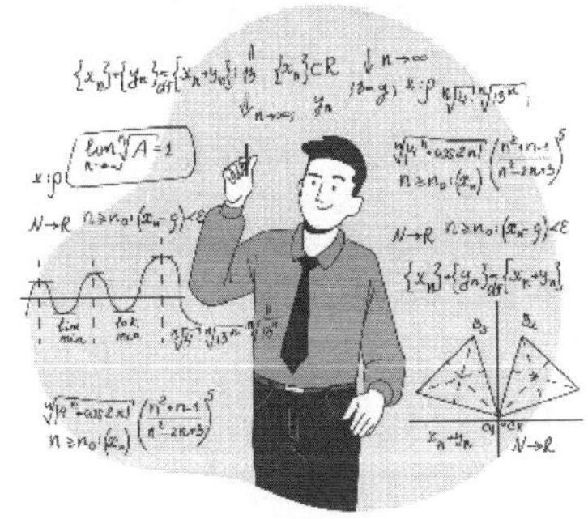

For any learning style, flashcards can be helpful. Organize the information so you can take advantage of spare moments to review. Underline key words or phrases. Use different colors for different categories. Mnemonic devices (such as creating a short list in which every item starts with the same letter) can also help with retention. Find what works best for you and use it to store the information in your mind most effectively and easily.

Secret Key 3: Practice the Right Way

Your success on test day depends not only on how many hours you put into preparing, but also on whether you prepared the right way. It's good to check along the way to see if your studying is paying off. One of the most effective ways to do this is by taking practice tests to evaluate your progress. Practice tests are useful because they show exactly where you need to improve. Every time you take a practice test, pay special attention to these three groups of questions:

- The questions you got wrong
- The questions you had to guess on, even if you guessed right
- The questions you found difficult or slow to work through

This will show you exactly what your weak areas are, and where you need to devote more study time. Ask yourself why each of these questions gave you trouble. Was it because you didn't understand the material? Was it because you didn't remember the vocabulary? Do you need more repetitions on this type of question to build speed and confidence? Dig into those questions and figure out how you can strengthen your weak areas as you go back to review the material.

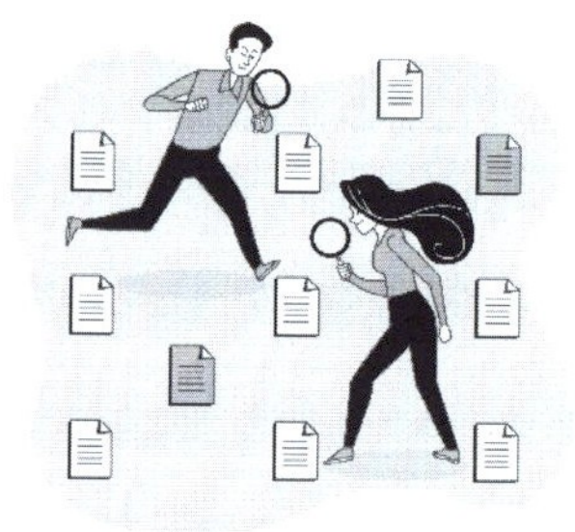

Additionally, many practice tests have a section explaining the answer choices. It can be tempting to read the explanation and think that you now have a good understanding of the concept. However, an explanation likely only covers part of the question's broader context. Even if the explanation makes perfect sense, **go back and investigate** every concept related to the question until you're positive you have a thorough understanding.

As you go along, keep in mind that the practice test is just that: practice. Memorizing these questions and answers will not be very helpful on the actual test because it is unlikely to have any of the same exact questions. If you only know the right answers to the sample questions, you won't be prepared for the real thing. **Study the concepts** until you understand them fully, and then you'll be able to answer any question that shows up on the test.

It's important to wait on the practice tests until you're ready. If you take a test on your first day of study, you may be overwhelmed by the amount of material covered and how much you need to learn. Work up to it gradually.

On test day, you'll need to be prepared for answering questions, managing your time, and using the test-taking strategies you've learned. It's a lot to balance, like a mental marathon that will have a big impact on your future. Like training for a marathon, you'll need to start slowly and work your way up. When test day arrives, you'll be ready.

Start with the strategies you've read in the first two Secret Keys—plan your course and study in the way that works best for you. If you have time, consider using multiple study resources to get different approaches to the same concepts. It can be helpful to see difficult concepts from more than one angle. Then find a good source for practice tests. Many times, the test website will suggest potential study resources or provide sample tests.

Practice Test Strategy

If you're able to find at least three practice tests, we recommend this strategy:

Untimed and Open-Book Practice

Take the first test with no time constraints and with your notes and study guide handy. Take your time and focus on applying the strategies you've learned.

Timed and Open-Book Practice

Take the second practice test open-book as well, but set a timer and practice pacing yourself to finish in time.

Timed and Closed-Book Practice

Take any other practice tests as if it were test day. Set a timer and put away your study materials. Sit at a table or desk in a quiet room, imagine yourself at the testing center, and answer questions as quickly and accurately as possible.

Keep repeating timed and closed-book tests on a regular basis until you run out of practice tests or it's time for the actual test. Your mind will be ready for the schedule and stress of test day, and you'll be able to focus on recalling the material you've learned.

Secret Key 4: Pace Yourself

Once you're fully prepared for the material on the test, your biggest challenge on test day will be managing your time. Just knowing that the clock is ticking can make you panic even if you have plenty of time left. Work on pacing yourself so you can build confidence against the time constraints of the exam. Pacing is a difficult skill to master, especially in a high-pressure environment, so **practice is vital**.

Set time expectations for your pace based on how much time is available. For example, if a section has 60 questions and the time limit is 30 minutes, you know you have to average 30 seconds or less per question in order to answer them all. Although 30 seconds is the hard limit, set 25 seconds per question as your goal, so you reserve extra time to spend on harder questions. When you budget extra time for the harder questions, you no longer have any reason to stress when those questions take longer to answer.

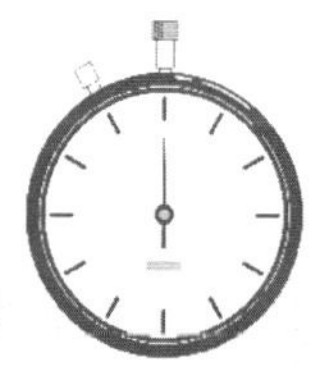

Don't let this time expectation distract you from working through the test at a calm, steady pace, but keep it in mind so you don't spend too much time on any one question. Recognize that taking extra time on one question you don't understand may keep you from answering two that you do understand later in the test. If your time limit for a question is up and you're still not sure of the answer, mark it and move on, and come back to it later if the time and the test format allow. If the testing format doesn't allow you to return to earlier questions, just make an educated guess; then put it out of your mind and move on.

On the easier questions, be careful not to rush. It may seem wise to hurry through them so you have more time for the challenging ones, but it's not worth missing one if you know the concept and just didn't take the time to read the question fully. Work efficiently but make sure you understand the question and have looked at all of the answer choices, since more than one may seem right at first.

Even if you're paying attention to the time, you may find yourself a little behind at some point. You should speed up to get back on track, but do so wisely. Don't panic; just take a few seconds less on each question until you're caught up. Don't guess without thinking, but do look through the answer choices and eliminate any you know are wrong. If you can get down to two choices, it is often worthwhile to guess from those. Once you've chosen an answer, move on and don't dwell on any that you skipped or had to hurry through. If a question was taking too long, chances are it was one of the harder ones, so you weren't as likely to get it right anyway.

On the other hand, if you find yourself getting ahead of schedule, it may be beneficial to slow down a little. The more quickly you work, the more likely you are to make a careless mistake that will affect your score. You've budgeted time for each question, so don't be afraid to spend that time. Practice an efficient but careful pace to get the most out of the time you have.

Secret Key 5: Have a Plan for Guessing

When you're taking the test, you may find yourself stuck on a question. Some of the answer choices seem better than others, but you don't see the one answer choice that is obviously correct. What do you do?

The scenario described above is very common, yet most test takers have not effectively prepared for it. Developing and practicing a plan for guessing may be one of the single most effective uses of your time as you get ready for the exam.

In developing your plan for guessing, there are three questions to address:

- When should you start the guessing process?
- How should you narrow down the choices?
- Which answer should you choose?

When to Start the Guessing Process

Unless your plan for guessing is to select C every time (which, despite its merits, is not what we recommend), you need to leave yourself enough time to apply your answer elimination strategies. Since you have a limited amount of time for each question, that means that if you're going to give yourself the best shot at guessing correctly, you have to decide quickly whether or not you will guess.

Of course, the best-case scenario is that you don't have to guess at all, so first, see if you can answer the question based on your knowledge of the subject and basic reasoning skills. Focus on the key words in the question and try to jog your memory of related topics. Give yourself a chance to bring the knowledge to mind, but once you realize that you don't have (or you can't access) the knowledge you need to answer the question, it's time to start the guessing process.

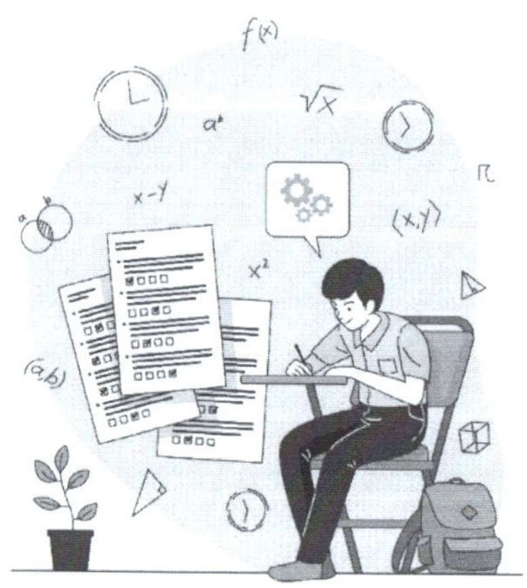

It's almost always better to start the guessing process too early than too late. It only takes a few seconds to remember something and answer the question from knowledge. Carefully eliminating wrong answer choices takes longer. Plus, going through the process of eliminating answer choices can actually help jog your memory.

Summary: Start the guessing process as soon as you decide that you can't answer the question based on your knowledge.

How to Narrow Down the Choices

The next chapter in this book (**Test-Taking Strategies**) includes a wide range of strategies for how to approach questions and how to look for answer choices to eliminate. You will definitely want to read those carefully, practice them, and figure out which ones work best for you. Here though, we're going to address a mindset rather than a particular strategy.

Your odds of guessing an answer correctly depend on how many options you are choosing from.

Number of options left	5	4	3	2	1
Odds of guessing correctly	20%	25%	33%	50%	100%

You can see from this chart just how valuable it is to be able to eliminate incorrect answers and make an educated guess, but there are two things that many test takers do that cause them to miss out on the benefits of guessing:

- Accidentally eliminating the correct answer
- Selecting an answer based on an impression

We'll look at the first one here, and the second one in the next section.

To avoid accidentally eliminating the correct answer, we recommend a thought exercise called **the $5 challenge**. In this challenge, you only eliminate an answer choice from contention if you are willing to bet $5 on it being wrong. Why $5? Five dollars is a small but not insignificant amount of money. It's an amount you could afford to lose but wouldn't want to throw away. And while losing $5 once might not hurt too much, doing it twenty times will set you back $100. In the same way, each small decision you make—eliminating a choice here, guessing on a question there—won't by itself impact your score very much, but when you put them all together, they can make a big difference. By holding each answer choice elimination decision to a higher standard, you can reduce the risk of accidentally eliminating the correct answer.

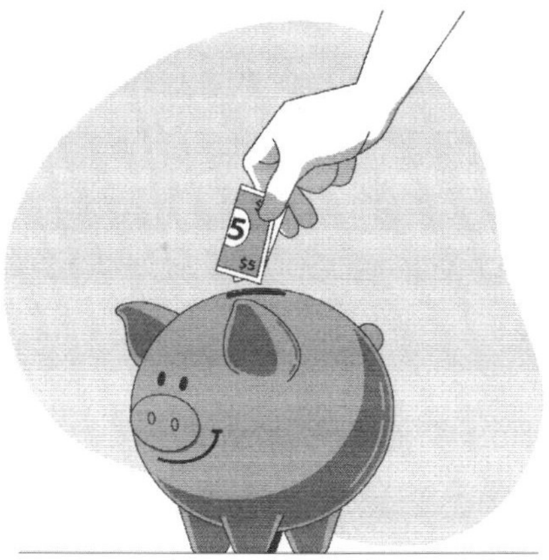

The $5 challenge can also be applied in a positive sense: If you are willing to bet $5 that an answer choice *is* correct, go ahead and mark it as correct.

Summary: Only eliminate an answer choice if you are willing to bet $5 that it is wrong.

Which Answer to Choose

You're taking the test. You've run into a hard question and decided you'll have to guess. You've eliminated all the answer choices you're willing to bet $5 on. Now you have to pick an answer. Why do we even need to talk about this? Why can't you just pick whichever one you feel like when the time comes?

The answer to these questions is that if you don't come into the test with a plan, you'll rely on your impression to select an answer choice, and if you do that, you risk falling into a trap. The test writers know that everyone who takes their test will be guessing on some of the questions, so they intentionally write wrong answer choices to seem plausible. You still have to pick an answer though, and if the wrong answer choices are designed to look right, how can you ever be sure that you're not falling for their trap? The best solution we've found to this dilemma is to take the decision out of your hands entirely. Here is the process we recommend:

Once you've eliminated any choices that you are confident (willing to bet $5) are wrong, select the first remaining choice as your answer.

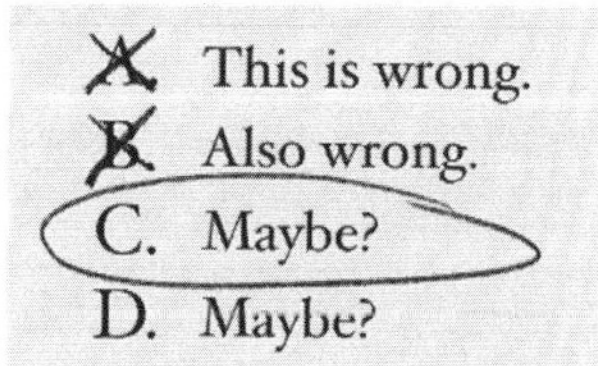

Whether you choose to select the first remaining choice, the second, or the last, the important thing is that you use some preselected standard. Using this approach guarantees that you will not be enticed into selecting an answer choice that looks right, because you are not basing your decision on how the answer choices look.

This is not meant to make you question your knowledge. Instead, it is to help you recognize the difference between your knowledge and your impressions. There's a huge difference between thinking an answer is right because of what you know, and thinking an answer is right because it looks or sounds like it should be right.

Summary: To ensure that your selection is appropriately random, make a predetermined selection from among all answer choices you have not eliminated.

Test-Taking Strategies

This section contains a list of test-taking strategies that you may find helpful as you work through the test. By taking what you know and applying logical thought, you can maximize your chances of answering any question correctly!

It is very important to realize that every question is different and every person is different: no single strategy will work on every question, and no single strategy will work for every person. That's why we've included all of them here, so you can try them out and determine which ones work best for different types of questions and which ones work best for you.

Question Strategies

✓ Read Carefully

Read the question and the answer choices carefully. Don't miss the question because you misread the terms. You have plenty of time to read each question thoroughly and make sure you understand what is being asked. Yet a happy medium must be attained, so don't waste too much time. You must read carefully and efficiently.

✓ Contextual Clues

Look for contextual clues. If the question includes a word you are not familiar with, look at the immediate context for some indication of what the word might mean. Contextual clues can often give you all the information you need to decipher the meaning of an unfamiliar word. Even if you can't determine the meaning, you may be able to narrow down the possibilities enough to make a solid guess at the answer to the question.

✓ Prefixes

If you're having trouble with a word in the question or answer choices, try dissecting it. Take advantage of every clue that the word might include. Prefixes can be a huge help. Usually, they allow you to determine a basic meaning. *Pre-* means before, *post-* means after, *pro-* is positive, *de-* is negative. From prefixes, you can get an idea of the general meaning of the word and try to put it into context.

✓ Hedge Words

Watch out for critical hedge words, such as *likely, may, can, often, almost, mostly, usually, generally, rarely,* and *sometimes.* Question writers insert these hedge phrases to cover every possibility. Often an answer choice will be wrong simply because it leaves no room for exception. Be on guard for answer choices that have definitive words such as *exactly* and *always.*

⊘ Switchback Words

Stay alert for *switchbacks*. These are the words and phrases frequently used to alert you to shifts in thought. The most common switchback words are *but, although*, and *however*. Others include *nevertheless, on the other hand, even though, while, in spite of, despite*, and *regardless of*. Switchback words are important to catch because they can change the direction of the question or an answer choice.

⊘ Face Value

When in doubt, use common sense. Accept the situation in the problem at face value. Don't read too much into it. These problems will not require you to make wild assumptions. If you have to go beyond creativity and warp time or space in order to have an answer choice fit the question, then you should move on and consider the other answer choices. These are normal problems rooted in reality. The applicable relationship or explanation may not be readily apparent, but it is there for you to figure out. Use your common sense to interpret anything that isn't clear.

Answer Choice Strategies

⊘ Answer Selection

The most thorough way to pick an answer choice is to identify and eliminate wrong answers until only one is left, then confirm it is the correct answer. Sometimes an answer choice may immediately seem right, but be careful. The test writers will usually put more than one reasonable answer choice on each question, so take a second to read all of them and make sure that the other choices are not equally obvious. As long as you have time left, it is better to read every answer choice than to pick the first one that looks right without checking the others.

⊘ Answer Choice Families

An answer choice family consists of two (in rare cases, three) answer choices that are very similar in construction and cannot all be true at the same time. If you see two answer choices that are direct opposites or parallels, one of them is usually the correct answer. For instance, if one answer choice says that quantity x increases and another either says that quantity x decreases (opposite) or says that quantity y increases (parallel), then those answer choices would fall into the same family. An answer choice that doesn't match the construction of the answer choice family is more likely to be incorrect. Most questions will not have answer choice families, but when they do appear, you should be prepared to recognize them.

⊘ Eliminate Answers

Eliminate answer choices as soon as you realize they are wrong, but make sure you consider all possibilities. If you are eliminating answer choices and realize that the last one you are left with is also wrong, don't panic. Start over and consider each choice again. There may be something you missed the first time that you will realize on the second pass.

⊘ Avoid Fact Traps

Don't be distracted by an answer choice that is factually true but doesn't answer the question. You are looking for the choice that answers the question. Stay focused on what the question is asking for so you don't accidentally pick an answer that is true but incorrect. Always go back to the question and make sure the answer choice you've selected actually answers the question and is not merely a true statement.

⊘ Extreme Statements

In general, you should avoid answers that put forth extreme actions as standard practice or proclaim controversial ideas as established fact. An answer choice that states the "process should be used in certain situations, if..." is much more likely to be correct than one that states the "process should be discontinued completely." The first is a calm rational statement and doesn't even make a definitive, uncompromising stance, using a hedge word *if* to provide wiggle room, whereas the second choice is far more extreme.

⊘ Benchmark

As you read through the answer choices and you come across one that seems to answer the question well, mentally select that answer choice. This is not your final answer, but it's the one that will help you evaluate the other answer choices. The one that you selected is your benchmark or standard for judging each of the other answer choices. Every other answer choice must be compared to your benchmark. That choice is correct until proven otherwise by another answer choice beating it. If you find a better answer, then that one becomes your new benchmark. Once you've decided that no other choice answers the question as well as your benchmark, you have your final answer.

⊘ Predict the Answer

Before you even start looking at the answer choices, it is often best to try to predict the answer. When you come up with the answer on your own, it is easier to avoid distractions and traps because you will know exactly what to look for. The right answer choice is unlikely to be word-for-word what you came up with, but it should be a close match. Even if you are confident that you have the right answer, you should still take the time to read each option before moving on.

General Strategies

⊘ Tough Questions

If you are stumped on a problem or it appears too hard or too difficult, don't waste time. Move on! Remember though, if you can quickly check for obviously incorrect answer choices, your chances of guessing correctly are greatly improved. Before you completely give up, at least try to knock out a couple of possible answers. Eliminate what you can and then guess at the remaining answer choices before moving on.

⊘ Check Your Work

Since you will probably not know every term listed and the answer to every question, it is important that you get credit for the ones that you do know. Don't miss any questions through careless mistakes. If at all possible, try to take a second to look back over your answer selection and make sure you've selected the correct answer choice and haven't made a costly careless mistake (such as marking an answer choice that you didn't mean to mark). This quick double check should more than pay for itself in caught mistakes for the time it costs.

⊘ Pace Yourself

It's easy to be overwhelmed when you're looking at a page full of questions; your mind is confused and full of random thoughts, and the clock is ticking down faster than you would like. Calm down and maintain the pace that you have set for yourself. Especially as you get down to the last few minutes of the test, don't let the small numbers on the clock make you panic. As long as you are on track by monitoring your pace, you are guaranteed to have time for each question.

⊘ Don't Rush

It is very easy to make errors when you are in a hurry. Maintaining a fast pace in answering questions is pointless if it makes you miss questions that you would have gotten right otherwise. Test writers like to include distracting information and wrong answers that seem right. Taking a little extra time to avoid careless mistakes can make all the difference in your test score. Find a pace that allows you to be confident in the answers that you select.

⊘ Keep Moving

Panicking will not help you pass the test, so do your best to stay calm and keep moving. Taking deep breaths and going through the answer elimination steps you practiced can help to break through a stress barrier and keep your pace.

Final Notes

The combination of a solid foundation of content knowledge and the confidence that comes from practicing your plan for applying that knowledge is the key to maximizing your performance on test day. As your foundation of content knowledge is built up and strengthened, you'll find that the strategies included in this chapter become more and more effective in helping you quickly sift through the distractions and traps of the test to isolate the correct answer.

Now that you're preparing to move forward into the test content chapters of this book, be sure to keep your goal in mind. As you read, think about how you will be able to apply this information on the test. If you've already seen sample questions for the test and you have an idea of the question format and style, try to come up with questions of your own that you can answer based on what you're reading. This will give you valuable practice applying your knowledge in the same ways you can expect to on test day.

Good luck and good studying!

Basic Sciences

Bacterial Infection in Surgical Patients

There are many factors that work together that can lead to the development of an infection in the surgical patient. First, the patient's overall health status should be taken into consideration, including any other chronic medical conditions from which they suffer. Poor nutritional status or a suppressed immune system leaves a patient more susceptible to developing an infection. The type of surgery that will be performed can have a higher risk of infection associated with it. Surgeries involving the GI tract can cause leaking of normal flora into the abdominal cavity which may cause infection. Certain bacteria are also more likely to cause an infection than others. For example, MRSA (methicillin-resistant *Staph. aureus*) is a very virulent strain of bacteria that can cause deadly infections. But even more common bacteria, such as *E. coli* and staph or strep can easily cause infections in the patient who has multiple co-morbidities or who has a compromised immune system.

Endogenous and Exogenous

Endogenous causes of infection are bacteria that are normally found in or on a person. This includes different variations of staphylococci which normally live on the skin. There are also bacteria that thrive within the body, such as *E. coli*, which is commonly found in the GI tract. Exogenous causes of infection are bacteria that are located away from the patient. This can include contamination of surgical instruments by bacteria or bacteria found on other inanimate objects that can potentially cause an infection in the patient.

Staphylococci Bacteria

Staphylococci bacteria are a very common cause of surgical site infections and have become more difficult to treat. *Staphylococcus epidermidis* is usually not treatable with methicillin, as well as some other common antibiotics. This can become an extremely dangerous infection if it is not treated with appropriate antibiotic therapy. Staphylococci bacteria are very common and many people, especially health care workers, can be colonized with the bacteria. This provides a ready source of bacteria available to infect patients. Most patients are infected through contaminated materials within the hospital or by direct transmission from health care workers. This particular type of bacteria is very resilient, even to standard cleaning products, so extra precaution should be given toward preventing infection in the patient through direct transmission. The most effective means of preventing transmission of organisms is through thorough hand washing before and after contact with a patient. Observing proper Universal Precaution standards also helps to prevent transmission of infectious agents.

Potential Complications of Infection

Staphylococci bacterial infections are most likely to begin with an incisional surgical site infection. These infections are painful when they begin. The initial appearance is redness around the incision, possibly with some warmth and a small amount of edema. If a discharge is present, it will most likely be thick and pale yellow in appearance. Recognition of the presence of an infection followed by appropriate antibiotic treatment is imperative at this stage to prevent progression of the infection to include organ or body cavity involvement, as well as the spread of the infection to a systemic state. There are certain types of staphylococcus bacteria that are more likely to cause severe infections. The infections can cause such severe conditions as toxic shock syndrome and sepsis. Toxic shock syndrome most often occurs from bacterial growth in material that is used for packing an area that is bleeding. Sepsis occurs as the infection spreads from the confined area of the surgical site throughout the body.

MRSA

MRSA stands for methicillin-resistant *Staphylococcus aureus*. It is a form of bacteria that is resistant to not only methicillin, but other medications within that class of antibiotics. This makes it very difficult to treat and can be life-threatening. Most patients acquire MRSA by contact with health care providers. It can live for several hours on the hands of staff members and is usually transmitted via that route. Unfortunately, many health care workers are already colonized with the bacteria and are not aware that they carry it. MRSA infections can affect wound infections, respiratory secretions, urine, and can even cause sepsis. In the surgical patient, it is most likely seen in an SSI. Once cultures return a diagnosis of MRSA, the patient should be placed in an isolation room on contact isolation precautions to prevent further transmission of the infection. Appropriate antibiotics should be given based on sensitivity results, though Vancomycin is the standard antibiotic given for treatment.

Streptococci Bacteria

Streptococci bacteria are common causes of infection. These are responsible for common bacterial respiratory infections in adults, ear infections in children, and severe infections that can be life threatening. There is now an immunization given to young children to help prevent common infections caused by strep bacteria. Group B strep is a bacterium that many people carry without even knowing it. Most pregnant women are tested for colonization with Group B strep before delivery to prevent serious infection in the infant after birth. Group A strep commonly causes skin infections, especially those associated with C-sections and other female reproductive system surgeries. Patients with diabetes and those with depressed immune systems are more susceptible to developing infections by Group A strep. Because strep is so common, antibiotic resistance has developed. The penicillin group of antibiotics is the most effective at treating strep, but has recently been found to be not as effective as in the past because of resistance.

Pseudomonas and Clostridia Bacteria

Pseudomonas is commonly found in warm, wet locations. It can cause a very serious infection in patients, especially in those with a depressed immune system, and can sometimes be found in the plastic tubing used with respirators. SSIs caused by Pseudomonas will cause a dark discharge that may be green or even light blue in color. It will also have a foul, stale odor different from other infections. Routine cleaning methods will kill Pseudomonas because it does not form spores.

Clostridia bacteria, on the other hand, are very difficult to kill and even some procedures used for sterilization will not eradicate the bacteria. Its resilience is due to the fact that it is capable of forming spores. This bacterium is associated with infections associated with tetanus exposure. It is also seen in wound infections that develop into gangrene and can involve loss of tissue or loss of a limb because of tissue death.

Enteric Bacilli Bacteria

The enteric bacilli bacteria are natural inhabits of the GI tract. Surgical infections involving these bacteria are often seen following procedures to the GI tract. This can range from an incisional SSI from direct contamination with *E. coli* bacteria to a serious infection involving the entire abdominal cavity caused by *Proteus* or *Enterobacter* as seen with peritonitis. Infections caused by enteric bacilli bacteria usually have a bad odor with a large amount of infectious discharge. The normal, healthy tissue is destroyed by these bacteria and is replaced with dead, necrotic tissue. Treatment of this infection should be started immediately once an infection is suspected to prevent the progression of the infection and prevent the death of any normal tissue. Infections by these bacteria have normally been treated with Vancomycin given intravenously, but antibiotic resistance has developed which has made the infections much harder to treat. This can be especially dangerous in those patients who have a compromised immune system or in the very young or elderly patients.

VRE

VRE stands for Vancomycin-resistant enterococcus infection. Vancomycin has commonly been the antibiotic of choice for treating difficult infections, such as MRSA, which has led to the development of resistance. This resistance has been seen somewhat with MRSA itself, but more often with the enterococcus bacteria. This is bacteria is also transmitted usually through contamination by health care providers. Surgical patients are more at risk for developing a VRE infection, as well as any patients who are hospitalized with a depressed immune system. Once culture results are available and confirm a diagnosis of VRE, the patient should be placed in an isolation room on contact isolation precautions to prevent further transmission of the infection. VRE can be very difficult to treat and multiple antibiotics are usually required, as well as the assistance of an infectious disease expert. VRE can be destroyed by normal disinfecting procedures, so careful hand washing is imperative to kill the bacteria on hands.

Tuberculosis

Tuberculosis is a serious respiratory illness that has increased in incidence in this country over the past few years. It is seen more frequently in patients who are homeless and those who have decreased immune systems. TB is transmitted through respiratory droplets. Exposure to the disease is evaluated with a PPD skin test. A positive response does not indicate that the person has TB, but rather the person has been exposed to the disease. A positive PPD is usually followed by a chest x-ray to check for the presence of any consolidated areas that may indicate a dormant TB infection. Prophylactic treatment may or may not be done with multiple antibiotics. Patients with TB must wear a specialized TB respiratory mask when being transported through public areas. The TB patient will be placed in a negative-pressure air flow room, on isolation. Strict respiratory/TB precautions should be followed to prevent transmission of the disease to other patients via health care workers.

Hepatitis A

Hepatitis A is contracted by exposure to contaminated feces or water. It is frequently seen in outbreaks where the central water source is contaminated or when people are eating food that has been prepared by someone who has the disease and transmits it through dirty hands. Risk factors for contracting the disease include living or vacationing in an area where the water is unsanitary. Engaging in close contact with an infected person who may be able to transfer the disease to a person through dirty hands, or eating foods that may be contaminated with dirty water or feces contamination all increase the risks of contracting hepatitis A. There is a vaccine available for hepatitis A that is given to those who will be traveling in areas in which the disease is prevalent. The disease can also be prevented by teaching proper hand washing techniques and by ensuring measures have been taken to provide water supplies that are sanitary. Avoiding raw seafood can also decrease the risk of contracting the disease.

Hepatitis B

Hepatitis B is spread through contact with infected blood or other bodily fluids. It can be sexually transmitted, acquired through sharing needles, or by contact with infected fluids when a person has an open sore or cut through which the virus can enter. Risk factors of developing hepatitis B include positions in which a person has the potential to be exposed to the virus by an infected individual. Health care workers can come in contact with blood or other bodily fluids that are infected with the virus. People with high risk behaviors such as IV drug abuse or multiple sexual partners place themselves at risk for acquiring hepatitis B. The prevention of hepatitis B is, obviously, avoiding the blood or body fluids of those individuals who are infected with the disease. This is not always possible, though. An immunization is available and is routinely given to those who are at risk. It is a series of three injections given over a 6-month time.

Hepatitis C

Hepatitis C is transmitted in the same in which hepatitis B is transmitted. Exposure to blood or body fluids of an infected individual can transmit the virus. A person may not develop symptoms and could become a carrier of the virus. Even though symptoms are not present, the virus can still be transmitted to uninfected individuals. Risk factors of developing hepatitis C include positions in which a person has the potential to be exposed to the virus by an infected individual. Health care workers can come in contact with blood or other bodily fluids that are infected with the virus. People with high risk behaviors such as IV drug abuse or multiple sexual partners place themselves at risk for acquiring hepatitis C. The prevention of hepatitis C is, obviously, avoiding the blood or body fluids of those individuals who are infected with the disease. There is no vaccine to prevent acquiring hepatitis C through exposure to infected fluids.

Hepatitis D

Hepatitis D cannot be acquired alone; rather, it occurs along with a hepatitis B infection. It is known that it must be transmitted through infected blood or body fluids, but little else is known because it has not been isolated on its own as a primary infection. Much about this disease is not known, such as when it is most likely to be transmissible. Risk factors of developing hepatitis D are the same as those for hepatitis B. Positions in which a person has the potential to be exposed to the virus by an infected individual increases the risk, such as health care workers being exposed to blood or other bodily fluids that are infected with the virus. Others at risk include IV drug abusers or those who practice unsafe sex. Vaccination to hepatitis B will prevent an individual from acquiring hepatitis D. Avoiding high risk behaviors and positions in which exposure to infected blood and body fluids can occur will also protect a person against the disease.

Hepatitis E

Hepatitis E is transmitted much the same way as hepatitis A. Contaminated water may contain the virus, especially in underdeveloped countries. It is also present in the feces of infected individuals and can be transmitted to others when proper hygiene is not performed. It is not, however, present in raw seafood or shellfish like hepatitis A can be. Risk factors include consuming contaminated water. Exposure to an individual with the disease who transmits it through their feces, usually by way of their hands, also can increase the risk of developing the disease. Prevention of the disease is by being very cautious about drinking water that may be contaminated, such as when traveling to an underdeveloped country. Individuals with hepatitis E can prevent transmission of the illness by carefully washing their hands after using the bathroom and before and after handling food. Unlike hepatitis A, there is no vaccine for the disease and most people recover without lasting effects.

Hepatitis G

Out of all of the hepatitis infections, the least amount of information is available about hepatitis G. It is transmitted through blood and is seen most frequently with hepatitis C. There may be other routes of transmission, but these are now known at this time. Risk factors for contracting hepatitis G include any situations that may cause a person to be exposed to infected blood. This can be a health care worker who provides direct patient care, an IV drug abuse, or a person who has had to receive blood transfusions. Many tests are performed on banked blood, but there is still a very small risk of contracting hepatitis or other blood-borne diseases through receiving blood. Preventing hepatitis G is accomplished much the same way as prevention of the other blood and body fluid hepatitis viruses, by avoiding situations in which exposure to blood infected with the virus may occur. There is no vaccine available to provide immunity to hepatitis G.

HIV

HIV is acquired by contact with the blood or body fluids of an infected individual. The virus can enter the uninfected individual through mucous membranes, through any open cuts or breaks in the skin, or through the eyes, as with a blood splash incident. The risk of transmission can be decreased by preventing exposure to a person's blood or other bodily fluids. This means wear gloves whenever there is the risk of exposure to body fluids, always use a condom during sexual activity, and avoid IV drug abuse, especially when needles are being shared. HIV can be transmitted from a mother to her baby while in utero, but babies usually test negative immediately after birth. Anti-retroviral medications can be given to the infant to prevent conversion to an HIV-positive state. Any individuals who have engaged in high risk behavior (IV drug abusers, homosexual males, those with multiple sex partners, or health care workers with frequent exposure to blood and body fluids) should be tested to assess their HIV status.

Herpes Simplex Viruses

Herpes simplex viruses can occur in two different forms. Type I involves an outbreak of lesions on the face or around the mouth. Type II causes lesions in the genital area. A person can have both types or may just have one type, but then can acquire the second type. Herpes simplex virus causes painful, blistering lesions that occur sporadically in outbreaks. There is no cure for either type of herpes, but there are medications available to help decrease the severity and frequency of outbreaks. Herpes simplex viruses are transmitted by direct exposure to the secretions from the lesions. With genital herpes, a person does not need to have the lesions present to transmit the disease. Contact with the secretions by hand can cause a form of herpes called herpetic whitlow which causes the lesions to form on the hands. Safe sexual practices and wearing gloves when there is a chance of exposure to herpetic lesions can prevent transmission.

Skin

The skin is the largest organ of the body and is necessary to provide protection of the underlying structures from infection, exposure to extreme temperatures, and to serve as a barrier allowing only certain substances to pass through it. The outermost layer of the skin is the epidermis and is composed of stratified squamous cells. It is the outermost barrier for protection. The second layer of skin cells forms the dermis. The dermis contains the blood and lymph supply for the skin, as well as nerves to perceive sensation and hair follicles. The sweat glands and sebaceous glands are located in certain areas of the body within the dermis. There are bacteria that normally live on the skin, called resident flora. It is kept at a healthy level through regulatory mechanisms of the body. When there is an alteration in the skin's integrity, such as a surgical incision, this bacterium could enter the body. If not properly controlled by the body's immune system, an infection could occur.

Necessities for Proper Wound Healing

Glucose and Fats

Glucose is the basic form of nutrition and energy for all of the body's cells. But not just glucose is necessary for wound healing. The glucose cannot be utilized by the cells if insulin is not present to carry it across the cell membrane (except in the brain where insulin is not required for glucose metabolism). Cells and tissues will die if they do not receive the proper nutrition provided by glucose and if insulin levels are not adequate to metabolize the glucose. Another effect on glucose metabolism is the process of gluconeogenesis. The liver can produce glucose from glucagon stores within the organ. If there is significant liver disease and damage, the liver cannot function appropriately to form this glucose. Fat cells have a primary role in formation of inflammatory cells. The inflammatory process is necessary to wound healing because of the presence of immune cells to fight off infection.

Proteins and Amino Acids

Amino acids are the building blocks of proteins and proteins are the fundamental ingredients necessary for tissue growth and development. If a patient has a low albumin, or protein level, there is a risk of poor healing. This impairs collagen synthesis and the ability of fibroblasts to function appropriately. The formation of blood supply to newly generated tissue can also be affected. Patients who are protein deficient have a higher likelihood of developing post-op wound complications. This includes wound dehiscence, or separation of the incision line, which can lead to infection. If protein levels are low, collagen synthesis can be impaired. Collagen provides most of the tensile strength in the wound to help form scar tissue. The maturation phase of wound healing, when scar tissue is remodeled and the wound obtains most of its strength, can also be impaired if protein levels are low. This can result in cosmetic changes in the incision and the resultant scar.

Vitamins A, C, and K

Vitamin A helps the macrophage cells to function within the wound area to participate in the inflammatory process. Vitamin A is also necessary for protein formation that helps to generate and strengthen tissues with collagen fibers. Vitamin C works mainly on collagen formation and collagen breakdown. This is essential in providing adequate tensile strength to the wound. In remodeling, or maturation, it is essential for vitamin C to breakdown some of the collagen to produce a smooth scar without contracture development. Vitamin K functions to help form some of the clotting factors necessary for hemostasis. If there is a deficiency in vitamin K, the patient can suffer hemorrhage with resultant wound seeping, bleeding, and hematoma formation. This can lead to a large seroma formation at the wound site, also. Patients with congenital deficiencies in vitamin K will need to receive vitamin K prior to and during surgery to control bleeding and prevent massive hemorrhage and development of hypovolemia.

Effects of Malnutrition on Wound Healing

A patient's overall nutritional status should be carefully assessed before surgery. Studies have shown that a patient who suffers from malnutrition is more likely to have complications following surgery with possible medical complications as well as complications of wound healing. When the body is placed under any type of stress, such as surgery, it responds by releasing cytoprotective substances that help to heal wounds and accommodate for any trauma that is suffered, such as blood loss or tissue damage. If a patient is malnourished, the body does not have the energy stores or appropriate protein levels and immune system response that are necessary to perform this function. This can result in medical complications, illness, an increased risk for infection, and poor wound healing. Patients who are malnourished may need to receive nutritional supplements to provide the adequate nutrients necessary for general good health and appropriate wound healing following surgery. A dietary consult may be necessary to formulate a nutrition plan for the patient.

Important Terms

Arthroplasty - Arthroplasty is the procedure in which an entire joint is replaced with a synthetic, movable model. This is typically seen with knee and hip replacements, as well as smaller joints such as the thumb.

Arthrodesis - Arthrodesis is performed when a joint replacement is not possible, but the joint needs to remain immobile in order to decrease pain. This commonly causes a fusion.

Osteotomy - Osteotomy is a procedure in which bones are cut and repositioned near a damaged joint. This is usually performed with severe arthritis.

Synovectomy - Synovectomy is the removal of the synovial lining that is located inside a joint. This lining is responsible for secreting synovial fluid which helps to lubricate the joint, but it can also be key in joint destruction. In auto-immune connective tissue disorders, such as rheumatoid arthritis, the synovial lining becomes destroyed by the body and a synovectomy can be performed to help decrease the pain.

Arthroscopy - Arthroscopy is minimally-invasive surgery using small incisions and scopes through which surgical procedures are performed.

Assessment Techniques

Patient History

The history is started with having the patient describe the course that has led up to their current illness. This would be the HPI, or history of present illness. All of the details of the illness should be described along with the time frame it has taken for these symptoms to develop. The past medical history, or PMH, is a listing of all illnesses for which the patient has been diagnosed. Surgical history includes all surgical procedures they have had in the past. Information should also be included regarding any complications they may have had from these procedures. The family history is important because it describes the medical conditions that other family members have suffered from. Chronic medical conditions of siblings, parents, aunts and uncles, and grandparents should be included. The social history describes the lifestyle factors that could affect a patient's illness. This is made up of the patient's marital status, number of children, type of work they do, and any tobacco/alcohol/recreational drugs they use.

Review of Systems

The review of systems, or ROS, includes any symptoms the patient may be having involving any of the body's major organ systems. This is recorded by starting at the head and working down, or cephalo-caudal. Start with the head, eyes, ears, nose, and throat, or HEENT. Include any pattern of headaches, changes in vision or hearing, any nasal or sinus symptoms, the presence of a sore throat or voice changes. Next is the respiratory system, or RESP, which includes cough, sputum production, or difficulty breathing. The cardiovascular system, or CV, includes chest pain, palpitations, swelling or edema in the extremities, or varicose veins. The gastrointestinal system, or GI, includes nausea, vomiting, diarrhea, constipation, abdominal pain, or change in bowel movements. The genitourinary, or GU, system includes changes in urination and normal sexual habits. For women, include menstrual and pregnancy history. The nervous system review includes any history of seizures. The skin history includes any rashes or chronic skin disorders. Psychiatric disorders, such as depression or anxiety, should also be reviewed.

Physical Exam

Inspection

Every part of the patient's body should be physically inspected. This is categorized by starting at the head and working down, or cephalo-caudally. The head shape and size should be assessed, including facial features and any changes in color of the skin. The eyes and oral mucosa should be assessed for any changes. The back and chest wall should be assessed for lung expansion that is equal bilaterally. The presence of upper body movement while breathing can indicate dyspnea. The extremities should be assessed for changes in color and edema or lesions. The abdomen should be inspected for any protrusions or changes in skin color. A patient may be guarding an area that is causing pain. The genital area should be inspected for any abnormalities or lesions. The presence of tremors of the extremities, including muscle twitches or tics, should be assessed. The skin should be inspected for any rashes, changes in color, or skin breakdown. The patient's emotional state may be evident by inspecting their facial expressions, or affect.

Percussion

Percussion is used to check the density of an area of the body. It is performed by placing the nondominant hand over the area to be examined. The middle finger is placed over the specific area to be percussed. The dominant middle finger is then used to tap sharply on the finger on the patient's body. This will produce a sound ranging from tympanic to flat. A tympanic sound is higher-pitched and hollow sounding. It is heard over areas that are filled with air, such as an empty stomach. A resonant sound is also heard over organs filled with air, but has a more echoing sound to it, such as over the lungs. An area that is overfilled with oxygen will sound hyper resonant and can be heard over the lungs in patients with emphysema. Dullness is heard over solid organs, such as the pancreas or liver. Flatness is heard over completely solid structures, such as bone or muscle.

Palpation

Palpation is the act of applying pressure, or feeling, an area of a patient's body to assess for any changes. The head can be palpated to assess for any nodules or bony changes. The neck and throat are palpated for enlarged lymph nodes. If a patient is having chest pain, the chest wall can be palpated for any reproducible pain. The extremities are palpated for any joint pain or the presence of nodules. Any areas of edema in the extremities should be palpated to check for pitting of the edema. The abdomen can be palpated for any enlargement of the organs and to assess for any reproducible pain. However, it is important to listen to, or auscultate, the abdomen before palpating. Palpating the abdomen can cause an increase in bowel sounds and the normal bowel sounds should be assessed first. Palpation is also used in the GU exam in males by performing a digital rectal exam and palpating the prostate gland for any nodules or irregular in size.

Auscultation

Auscultation is listening to an area of the body using a stethoscope. This is used over the heart to assess for normal heart sounds (lub dub, or S1 and S2). It is also used during the cardiovascular exam to assess for heart murmurs or extra heart sounds (S3). The chest wall should be auscultated over the upper areas on both sides and along the left sternal border and the left ribs. The carotid arteries can be auscultated for a bruit which represents a narrowing of a vessel. The lungs are auscultated to detect normal breath sounds. The lungs should be auscultated on each side of the upper lung fields, the lower lung fields and the sides to fully evaluate the patient for any wheezing, crackles, or pleural rubs. The abdomen is auscultated for bowel sounds and any bruits that can be detected over the abdominal aorta and renal arteries. The abdomen should be auscultated before it is palpated or percussed to prevent causing an increase in bowel sounds.

Orthopedic Patients

Patient History

Besides the regular past medical history, surgical history, and family history that is taken on every patient, more focused questions should be asked regarding the nature of the patient's problem. This would include what is wrong and any associated symptoms. These symptoms can include pain, swelling, immobility, difficulty moving, effects of the pain on their ADLs, and any aggravating or relieving factors. The time frame in which this has occurred should be included. If an injury is the cause of the patient's current symptoms and the reason for surgery, be sure to clarify what happened. Take a careful of the patient's past medical history to assess for any conditions that may impair the healing process or may place the patient at risk during surgery. These include diabetes, heart disease, vascular disease, and dementia. Some patients may require surgical clearance from specialists, such as cardiologists, pulmonologists, or vascular specialists, before surgery can be performed.

Physical Exam

The physical exam begins with inspection. The area of injury or the surgical site should be examined for any edema, erythema, or gross deformity (such as with a traumatic fracture). With some conditions, there may be no physical change noted at all. When palpating the area, avoid applying pressure over a fractured bone to avoid excessive pain. It is important, however, to thoroughly assess the pulses in an affected limb to ensure that vascular damage has not occurred during an injury. The patient should also be assessed for any sensory deficits which may occur with nerve damage. There are multiple maneuvers to perform depending on the patient's injury. Tests such as the anterior and posterior drawer signs with knee ligament injury are specialized for specific conditions and should be performed if appropriate. Simply walking a patient walk if there is a lower limb problem can reveal a great deal of information.

Diagnostic Studies

Regular pre-operative studies will be performed, depending on the facility's requirements. These could include a chest x-ray and EKG. Laboratory tests will include a basic metabolic profile, CBC, urinalysis to rule out infection, and possibly coagulation studies. Other diagnostic studies to be performed will be specific to the scheduled surgery. At minimum, an x-ray of the affected limb will be necessary.

Usually, an MRI is performed, or if contraindicated, a CT is performed. These are often necessary to have in the operating room to carefully assess joint spaces for prosthesis placement. Other specialized testing that may be performed includes Doppler ultrasound testing to assess blood flow in an affected limb. This will ensure that a DVT is not present and that pressures within a vessel are normal. If there is a concern for nerve damage, an EMG/NCV (electromyogram/nerve conduction velocity) test may be performed. This is the diagnostic test of choice for diagnosing peripheral nerve disorders such as carpal tunnel syndrome or ulnar neuropathy.

Review Video: EKG Rhythms - Reading the Graph
Visit mometrix.com/academy and enter code: 872282

Cardiac Patients

Patient History

The patient should be questioned about any prior cardiovascular surgeries they have undergone in the past. Cardiac bypass grafting requires that another vein in the body, usually the greater saphenous vein in the leg, is harvested for use as the graft. If the patient has had previous bypass surgery, or if they have had vein stripping procedures performed on this vein in the past, another vessel may be chosen. This could include the lesser saphenous vein or even an artery, such as the radial artery. This not used as often now, but the patient should be assessed for adequate blood flow in the upper extremity and asked if they ever have symptoms such as color changes, coldness, or numbness in the hand or arm. Information should be gathered from the patient regarding their current medication regimen. This would include all anticoagulant medications such as aspirin, Plavix, or Coumadin. Some vitamins and herbal supplements can also pose a risk for increased bleeding during surgery, such as vitamin E and garlic.

Pre-Operative Testing

Basic screening laboratory testing will be done before cardiac surgery. This included a CBC, chemistry panel, LFTs, coagulation studies, urinalysis, chest x-ray, and EKG. These are the same tests generally performed before most surgeries. However, specific cardiac testing may need to be performed before a patient undergoes major cardiac surgery. An echocardiogram provides an ultrasound image of the heart to evaluate function and valve function. This may be necessary to assess the ejection fraction, which is the percentage measurement that indicates the amount of blood that is ejected from the heart with each beat. An echocardiogram can also show back flow of blood when a malfunctioning valve is present. Cardiac catheterization will be performed before cardiac bypass surgery and determines the amount of cardiac artery occlusion that is present. This test is frequently performed in patients with signs of cardiac ischemia. It can also be performed to place cardiac stents and avoid arterial bypass surgery.

Preoperative Physical Exam

The extremity to be used for vein or artery harvesting should be carefully examined for any signs of decreased blood flow. If the radial artery is to be used, an Allen's test should be performed in which both the radial and ulnar arteries are compressed until the hand appears pale. Pressure is released from the ulnar artery to ensure it is patent and provides adequate blood flow to the hand. The radial artery can also be tested for patency by releasing the pressure on it to check if blood flow returns to the hand. A careful heart and lung exam should be performed to assess for any abnormal breath sounds or the presence of a murmur, gallop, or rub. The carotid arteries should be auscultated for bruits. This is especially important when the internal mammary artery is being considered for use because this could indicate decreased blood flow to that artery.

Laboratory Tests Performed Before Surgery

Most medical facilities have established criteria regarding lab tests that need to be completed prior to a patient having surgery. These may be simple, routine tests, but some patients may require more specific, specialized testing done before going to the OR. A basic metabolic panel, or chemistry panel, will be done. This will measure electrolytes, such as sodium, potassium, chloride, carbon dioxide, BUN, creatinine, and glucose levels. Liver function tests may be done to assess liver function. A complete blood count (CBC) will be done to check for an elevated white blood cell count before surgery, as well as assess the patient's red blood cell count, hemoglobin, and hematocrit levels. This can provide a baseline to determine if the patient is becoming anemic following surgery. A urinalysis (U/A) may be done to check for any underlying urinary tract infection. A chest x-ray (CXR) may also be performed to ensure the patient does not have underlying respiratory disease. Depending on the patient's age and co-morbidities, an EKG may also be performed.

Assessment for Risk of Hemorrhage

A complete blood count (CBC) should be done pre-operatively to assess the patient's baseline hemoglobin and hematocrit levels. The red blood cell (RBC) and white blood cell (WBC) counts are also important. A patient may have a slow bleeding vessel within the surgical wound that is not visible immediately post-op. A steady decline in the hemoglobin level can point to a possible internal cause for the bleeding. The CBC will also include a platelet count. A decreased number of platelets can affect blood clotting. Liver function tests (LFTs) should be performed to assess the patient's overall liver function. Several clotting factors and proteins are produced by the liver and any liver damage could affect this. Coagulation studies, such as a prothrombin time (PT), international normalization ratio (INR), and partial thromboplastin time (PTT) should be assessed to evaluate for any coagulopathies. This is especially important in patients who have been taking heparin or Coumadin before surgery.

Informed Consent Document

The informed consent is a legal document that is completed prior to surgery. Its function is to describe a surgical procedure, along with risks and benefits. All of the information in the informed consent needs is fully explained to the patient and it is signed by the operating physician and the patient, or patient representative. It is witnessed by another person who will not be involved in the surgery, but not a friend or family member of the patient. The informed consent clearly explains, in layman's terms, the procedure that will be performed. Any potential risks should be explained and included in writing. These risks include bleeding, incidence of infection, potential for any permanent nerve or organ damage, or even death. The informed consent should be reviewed with the patient when they are fully alert, before any medications have been given, and when their anxiety level is lowest. This is not always possible in an emergency situation, and the patient's decision maker will need to complete the informed consent.

Pre-Anesthesia Assessment

A thorough history and physical exam should be performed on the patient before anesthesia is administered. The history should include all previous surgeries the patient has had, including any reactions to anesthesia that have occurred in the past. A medical history should be obtained, paying special attention to any cardiac or respiratory illnesses the patient may suffer from. The physical exam should include a thorough heart and respiratory exam to assess for any abnormalities. Any physical changes in the patient that may interfere with the induction of anesthesia should also be recorded. Patients who are very obese or those who suffer from musculoskeletal disease affecting the cervical spine may be difficult to intubate because of limited mobility. It is very important to know when the patient last ate. Anesthesia may cause expulsion of the stomach contents and could lead to aspiration. Special precautions need to be taken if surgery cannot be avoided in the patient who ate within the past 8 hours.

Contributing Factors to Bleeding During or After Surgery

The type of surgery performed is the most important contributing factor to the development of bleeding during or after surgery. Certain areas of the body are more vascular than others, such as the brain, heart, spleen, and liver. Surgeries performed on these areas of the body may result in intra-operative hemorrhage or postoperative hemorrhage if there is continued seeping of blood from vessels in the area. The patient's coagulability status is also a factor. Patients who have been treated with anticoagulants before surgery, and in an emergency situation, were not able to stop these medications in time for surgery, are at risk for developing intraoperative bleeding. The use of certain anticoagulants, such as heparin, may result in postop bleeding. Patients who undergo surgery to remove a tumor may develop intra-operative bleeding. Certain types of tumor tend to be very vascular. Disruption of this blood flow with severing of the vessels could result in excessive bleeding.

Integrated Patient Record

The integrated patient record serves as a combined record that includes the documentation from many different specialties. For example, the physician's notes will be included as well as the nursing notes. The CRNFA pre-op and post-op notes will be included as well as physical therapy documentation. The advantage of an integrated patient record is that a healthcare provider can use one patient record to access the information on a patient to help guide the treatment plan. For example, if a patient is going for surgery in the morning, the CRNFA can look at the nurse's notes and find out the patient was having a lot of anxiety the evening before because of apprehension regarding surgery. Lab values in the chart can also be available the morning of surgery to ensure there are no medical contraindications for surgery. By accessing these records, for example, the CRNFA can adjust the treatment plan as necessary to provide more comfort to the patient, or prepare for any potential complications due to abnormal lab results.

Evaluation of Patient Care

The ongoing evaluation of care provided to the patient is an excellent learning process which benefits the healthcare professional as well as the patient. Whether medical care or nursing care is evaluated, the outcome will be helpful in guiding the direction for the future care of each patient. For example, specific medical treatments that are used on patients can be evaluated by both the nurses who administer these treatments as well as the physicians ordering them. The decision can then be made to continue with the treatment that has been started, or to change the treatment plan to produce a more beneficial effect for the patient. Nursing interventions and treatments can also be evaluated and reviewed to determine their effectiveness in achieving the goal set forth. This information gathered in reassessing the treatment plan can then be used not just for this patient, but possibly for other patients in the future as well.

Individual Clinical Decision Making

Nurses should be encouraged to develop their patient assessment skills to the fullest in order to use these skills in clinical decision making with the patient. Having a nurse who is comfortable, confident, and knowledgeable in assessing a patient and then utilizing critical thinking skills is advantageous to the patient. Physicians also rely heavily upon the nursing staff to provide accurate, knowledgeable information regarding a patient if they are not present. Nurses see their patients regularly during the shift and can access the patient for any change in symptoms or signs of distress. Excellent clinical decision-making skill will enable the nurse to make the right decision when choosing the appropriate intervention for a patient. This also helps to instill a sense of self-confidence, self-accomplishment, and accountability in the nurse. The other medical staff will appreciate the accurate decision-making skills of the nurse which will add to their standing as a trusted, respected member of the medical team.

Intraoperative Knowledge

Asepsis

Asepsis is the practice of performing a specific act or procedure without the presence of an infective organisms or substances that may compromise the sterility of the area. This term can be applied to the state of the surgical field which must remain free or germs and requires that aseptic technique be used when working within this field. Florence Nightingale was the first known nurse to promote the practice of asepsis when providing patient care. She had found that more frequent care that was given to keeping patient's free of germ contamination, especially surgical sites, resulted in a fewer number of infections. Johns Hopkins University was the first institution to utilize a standard surgical scrub in place of rinsing hands with acid before surgery. They also instituted the practice of wearing sterile surgical gowns. The Goodyear Company worked closely with one of the surgeons at Johns Hopkins to develop rubber gloves to be worn in surgery.

Surgical Site Infections

The following are the different types of surgical site infections (SSI):

- Incisional – This type of SSI only affects the incision. It is a skin infection and is usually easily treated with appropriate oral antibiotic therapy.
- Superficial incisional – This type of SSI affects the skin at the incision site along with the subcutaneous tissue immediately surrounding the incision. It may be treated with oral antibiotics or may require IV antibiotic therapy. If not responsive to antibiotic therapy, this may require incision and drainage.
- Deep incisional – This type of SSI not only involves the incision and the subcutaneous tissue surrounding the incision, but also extends deeper into the connective tissue and muscle in the area. This can be quite extensive and can cause significant tissue damage in the area if left untreated. Antibiotics given IV are necessary and the infection usually requires surgical treatment as well.
- Organ/space – This type of SSI is an internal infection that does not involve the incision itself. Rather, this occurs within the body at the site where surgery occurred and can involve abscess formation or extensive organ involvement.

Risk Factors

Risk factors for the development of a surgical site infection (SSI) generally fall into two major categories: those factors that the patient brings with them to surgery and those that are out of the patient's control within the operating room. Patient risk factors include their overall health condition along with the presence of any co-morbidities. Social habits, such as smoking, drinking, or drug use, can increase the risk of an SSI. Socioeconomic factors such as poor living conditions, poor nutrition, and lack of access to healthcare can increase infection risks. The conditions within the operating room can directly affect the patient's risk of developing an SSI. These include the sterility procedures and maintenance of a sterile field during surgery. Proper operative site preparation, including hair removal and site prep, can affect whether the patient develops an SSI. Other factors include the use of antibiotics during surgery, the length of surgery, and the type of wound closure that is used.

Perioperative Antibiotic Use

The three main factors to consider when using perioperative antibiotics include when the antibiotic should be given, which antibiotic to use at what dose, and when it is appropriate to use antibiotics. Studies have shown that the most appropriate time to administer antibiotics is approximately 1 hour before surgery begins. The effectiveness of prophylactic antibiotic therapy decreases once the surgical incision is made and the initial dose of antibiotics should not be given after that time. A broad-spectrum antibiotic that will kill the bacteria commonly responsible for causing SSIs should be used. This is usually a cephalosporin unless this contraindicated because of direct allergy or penicillin allergy. Vancomycin is usually used in those cases. This should be given in a large dose, not low dose, to provide appropriate coverage. Many surgeons use antibiotics for all invasive procedures, but the type of surgery should also be considered. For surgeries that have a very low risk of infection, the risks and benefits of antibiotic use should be considered based on the patient.

Preparation of Skin for Surgery

Preparation of the surgical site varies depending on the type of surgery, the hospital procedures, and the surgeon's preference. It is important to prep the site so that bacteria will be killed, the environment will not be favorable for regrowth of bacteria, the patient will be free of harm, and preserving patient privacy. The skin is first cleansed with a cleansing formula, using a circular pattern, going from dirty areas to clean. The antiseptic is then used, such as iodine. It is applied using sponges held with forceps or using special sponge applicators that are included in a prep kit. This is also applied by starting at the middle of the area where the incision will be made, and cleaning out from the middle point. Antiseptic should be applied at least twice. The prep should be completed quickly to prevent contamination. Special care should be given to prevent irritation of skin that will not be part of the surgical field because antiseptic solutions may be caustic to the skin.

The purpose of cleansing the skin before surgery is to remove as much of the resident flora as possible, as well as clean the area of any dirt or oil that may be present. The skin will not be sterile during surgery, but a protective film that is sterile will be adhered over it through which the surgical incision is made. Hair on the skin can contain many different types of bacteria, as well as dirt and oil. Depending on the surgical site and the surgeon's preference, all hair in the area of the incision may be removed using clippers or a razor. Care needs to be given, though, to prevent any nicking or cuts in the skin because they can later serve as an area through which bacteria can enter the area around the surgical site and cause an infection. There is ongoing research regarding the safety of removing hair from the surgical site because of the risk of infection in the area.

Cleansing Agents

The two most common bacteria causing surgical site infections are *Staphylococcus aureus* and *Staphylococcus epidermidis*. There are several agents used to cleanse the skin prior to surgery that are effective at controlling the growth of these organisms. Iodine or iodine compounds are commonly used and provide a stained outline of the area on which surgery will occur. It can cause irritation of the skin and any excess liquid should be absorbed to avoid prolonged exposure to the iodine in areas outside the surgical site. Some patients have severe allergic reactions to iodine and they should not be cleansed with this. Patients with an allergy to seafood should also not be treated with iodine. Chlorhexidine gluconate can also be used to cleanse the surgical site. It is less likely to cause skin irritation like iodine, but is effective for only about 6 hours. Ethyl alcohol has limited use because it can cause damage to internal tissues and mucous membranes. It is also very flammable and is not used very often.

Precautions

Standard precautions are guidelines that should be followed to prevent exposure to blood or body fluids from all patients. These provide standards for protective gear to be worn, disposable of sharps, cleaning body fluid spills, and isolation room guidelines. Transmission-based precautions are used when a specific disease state is known. They are guidelines followed to prevent transmission of this disease. An example of this would be the isolation room requirements and protective gear used when caring for patients with tuberculosis. Airborne precautions outline the procedures to prevent transmission of diseases which are transmitted through the air. This includes any special masks that should be worn. An example of this is chicken pox (Varicella virus). Droplet precautions outline what guidelines should be followed to prevent transmission of diseases which are transmitted by exposure to respiratory droplets. An example of this is tuberculosis. Contact precautions are followed when caring for patients who have diseases that are transmitted through contact with the individual. An example of this is a MRSA skin infection.

Drapes

Sterile drapes are used to ensure an aseptic field is maintained in the area surrounding the surgical site. Each hospital and surgery center will use its preferred type of drape. Reusable drapes are made out of cotton and are very breathable. They can be washed and sterilized, but are only able to go through this process a certain number of times before they must be discarded. It can become very costly for a hospital to use this type of drapes because of the work involved with preparing the drapes for re-use. Single-use drapes are disposable and very light. They are easy to work with many have certain qualities that help to prevent bacteria from adhering to them. They are also fire-proof and moisture-proof. This type of drape is not biodegradable and can pose a problem with the bulk of excess waste to be disposed of. Cost can also be an issue for an item that is going to be thrown away.

Measures to Maintain Sterile Surgical Field

Draping should be done in an efficient manner to minimize the amount of contact the RN First Assistant will have with it. A sense of awareness during draping is very important to prevent unintentional contamination of the sterile drape. Care should be taken in preventing any contamination of the gloves or gown worn by the CRNFA who is draping the patient. The drape is left folded out of the package and opened so that the ends are hanging off the bed. The section of drape that falls below the edge of the bed is considered contaminated. Care should be taken to prevent leaning over the patient while applying the drapes. The drape should not be held down, but should remain within the line of vision and held above the waist. If there is any question whether a drape has become contaminated, it should be replaced. It is smarter to dispose of an unused drape rather than risk exposing the surgical site to bacteria that could potentially cause a serious infection.

Draping Techniques

Draping begins with isolating the surgical site. This is accomplished by using surgical towels around the four sides of the location where the incision will be made. These towels can be reusable or disposable. Reusable drapes are held in place using clamps, while disposable towels are self-adhesive. Instead of using surgical towels, an incise drape may be used. This is a large drape that requires two people for proper placement. A fenestrated sheet is placed over the patient after the surgical towel or incise drape are in place. The fenestrated sheet is designed especially for specific surgical sites. The opening in the sheet is large enough for the surgical procedure to be performed, but not too large that an excess area of non-operative, or unsterile, area is exposed. The sheet does not to be large enough, though, that there is extension of the sterile area outside the actual surgical field to avoid contamination from unsterile areas.

Anesthesia

History and Evolution

It was not until half-way through the 19th century that anesthesia was used during surgery. Before this time, patients often did not survive surgery and would die of shock or hemorrhage, among other complications. In the mid-1800s patients were given ether for anesthesia, preceded by drinking large quantities of whiskey to help with inducing unconsciousness. Shortly after this, nitrous oxide was invented, which is frequently used today for anesthesia. As more research was done, more gases became available that could be safely used to induce sedation. Other medications were approved for to be used for spinal anesthesia and to provide local anesthesia. Research is currently being conducted to improve anesthesia and develop new ways to administer anesthesia to provide more pain relief for the patient in a safe manner. Other studies are being conducted to judge the effectiveness of administering analgesics to patients prior to surgery in an effort to control pain before they are woken up after anesthesia administration.

Types of Anesthesia

Rapid sequence intubation is performed by first administering an IV medication that will sedate the patient. Another medication is given as a paralyzing agent to prevent involuntary movements of the body. The endotracheal tube is inserted between the vocal cords and a cuff around the tube is inflated to prevent its movement. Regional anesthesia provides anesthesia to a specific area. An example of this is a Bier block used to anesthetize the arm and is frequently used in carpal tunnel and ulnar nerve surgeries. Epidural/spinal anesthesia involves injecting anesthetizing medication into the epidural space of the spine to block sensation of the lower extremities. It is most commonly known of for its use in labor and delivery. Monitored anesthesia is also known as conscious sedation or twilight sleep. It provides anesthesia without completely sedating the patient. This is commonly used during colonoscopy procedures. Local anesthesia involves anesthetizing a specific small area. It is used for small procedures, such as I & D of an abscess or when suturing a laceration.

Safety Concerns When Positioning Anesthetized Patient

One of the priorities during anesthesia is to ensure the patient is safe and free from injury. First, the patient should be on the table in a way that there is no risk he or she will fall off during surgery. When a great deal of force is continually applied to the body's pressure points, joint or nerve damage can occur. This may be transient or permanent. The most common nerves that are injured are those that make up the brachial plexus near the axillae. This is especially true when the arm is extended to the side and the head is facing the opposite direction. Blood flow to an area can be inhibited when pressure is applied for an extended period of time. This can lead to tissue damage at the site of vessel compression as well as damage to the area distal to this site. This can lead to necrosis of the tissue.

Monitoring Patient During Surgery

The patient's cardiovascular status will be continually monitored throughout surgery. This is accomplished by EKG monitoring and blood pressure. Special venous and arterial lines may also be inserted to closely monitor intravascular pressure. The patient's respiratory status will also be closely monitored. Pulse oximetry can be used to monitor the oxygenation status and simple inspection of the patient's skin can show cyanosis if there is a decline in circulating oxygen. The function of the respiratory system can also be monitored by monitoring the tidal volume and through other specialized monitoring systems. Temperature will be monitored with an esophageal stethoscope or by direct measurements of the skin temperature. Urine output can be monitored with a urinary catheter. The amount of blood the patient loses during surgery is measured in a collection device connected to the suction unit. The amount of blood lost during surgery can also be estimated by assessing the sponges that are used to absorb lost blood.

Operating Room Lighting

There are usually two lights in the operating room. Once the patient is on the operating room, but before they have been given any anesthesia, the operating table should be positioned so that one light is shining down on their head and one on their feet. This allows the lights to be in a position so that they can be moved during surgery to illuminate just about any surface of the patient's body. The operating room lights have handles that are covered with sterile covers so that they can be manipulated during surgery. Generally, the lights are always positioned above the patient to shine down on the surgical site. In surgeries involving the head and mouth, the light may be positioned behind the surgeon and CRNFA and angled to shine up into the surgical site. With some deep surgeries or surgeries that take place within a small area, a small light may be attached to the surgeon's head to shine down in the area where he is focused.

Equipment Positioning Techniques

One of the roles of the RN First Assistant is to ensure surgeries are completed in a timely manner and as efficiently as possible. Though speed is the most important quality of the surgeon and CRNFA, some basic preparation can contribute to decreasing the time in which the patient is anesthetized and contribute to a shorter surgery time. Most RN First Assistants will work with the same surgeon(s) over and over again. This helps to learn the surgeon's preferences with patient positioning and OR set up preferences. A right-handed surgeon will prefer to be on the patient's right during most procedures. The table should be at a level to avoid excess elevation of the arms or excess bending at the waist which can cause muscle fatigue and interfere with fine motor control. If it is necessary to operate on an area of the body that is very deep, such as with an anterior approach to spine surgery, the table should be slightly lower to facilitate extension of the arms.

Incisions

Standard Midline Incision

The standard midline incision is made with the scalpel perpendicular to patient. It extends down the middle of the lower abdomen from just below the umbilicus to just above the pubis. It is a very common incision because it provides adequate visualization of the contents of the lower abdomen. The linea alba is a vertical line of hypopigmented skin that may be difficult to see in some patients. It is directly below the umbilicus. An incision made through this line generally has few complications than incision in other areas of the abdomen. The section of the linea alba covering the abdominal organs distal to the umbilicus has very little blood supply and no nerve supply, so blood loss and pain are decreased. The standard midline incision can also be lengthened if necessary during surgery to provide better visualization of the surgical site. There is a risk of incisional hernias in an incision that is made above the umbilicus and this should be considered when suturing the incision after surgery.

Rectus Incision

The different types of rectus incisions are made in or around the rectus muscle which runs vertically over the middle of the abdomen from above the umbilicus to the pubic area. A rectus incision is termed paramedian when it is made vertically in a position lateral to the umbilicus, but median to the edge of the rectus muscle border. Pararectus incisions are made vertically over the left or right lateral border of the muscle. Transrectus incisions are made through the midline of the muscle at its thickest point. Transrectus incisions are generally not used because of the amount of bleeding that is involved when an incision is made through the thickest portion of the muscle. The nerves that control the rectus muscle enter the area through the lateral borders, so there is risk of nerve damage with a pararectus incision. The paramedian is used more often than the other rectus incisions because it avoids the nerves over the lateral border and less bleeding than with transrectus incisions.

Kocher Oblique Incision

The Kocher oblique incision is made on an angle extending from the midline laterally. It runs just underneath the lower ribs. When made on the right side, it is commonly used for removal of the gallbladder. The same incision can be made on the left side, also, to access the pancreas or spleen. An incision can also be made with the superior ends meeting at the midline. This provides access to all of the vital abdominal organs with very clear visualization. This is preferred over paramedian or midline incisions because it provides not only a broad horizontal area for visualization, but vertical visualization as well. Many cholecystectomies, or gallbladder removals, are done using a laparoscopic approach, that this incision is not used as frequently for this procedure. When it is used, accessing the gallbladder may take some time because of the care involved with passing through the rectus muscle fibers.

McBurney Oblique Incision

A McBurney oblique incision is used when the appendix must be removed through an open incision instead of laparoscopically. It is made in the right lower quadrant of the abdomen at a 45-degree angle extending from the lateral point superiorly to the medial point inferiorly. The incision is made at an angle running parallel with the external oblique muscle fibers. This incision is usually about 4-5 inches long. There is less abdominal weakness following an appendectomy with this type of incision because the angle at which it is made allows for the muscle fibers to be separated rather than severed. This helps the patient to heal faster following surgery with decreased complaints of pain. The angle at which this incision is made also allows for room to completely visualize the appendix and surrounding structures in order to efficiently perform the surgery. The McBurney oblique incision is used when the appendix has ruptured or if a laparoscope approach is not possible.

Transverse Incision

The transverse incision is made horizontally and extends through the abdominal wall. It can be made at any level in the abdomen and on the left side, right side, or extending across the entire abdomen. Though it provides access to a wide area of the abdomen, there is not a lot of visualization provided for structures that are far superior or inferior in the abdomen simultaneously. This incision provides fewer potential complications than a vertical incision because the superficial nerves and vessels in the abdomen do not need to be transected. This helps to reduce the post-op pain while healing occurs which can shorten the convalescence period for most patients. A transverse incision can also blend with the natural skin creases and folds over time to reduce the amount of scarring the patient will have following surgery. Vertical incision scars tend to have a widened appearance after healing has occurred.

Lower Oblique Incision

The lower oblique incision is made on an angle down low in the abdomen and extending somewhat laterally. It is used to access the kidneys and major urological organs, as well as some of the major blood vessels, such as the abdominal aorta. There is significant muscle dissection with this incision and the surgeon must penetrate the muscles located on the patient's flank. There has been significant research over the past few years with utilizing this approach to provide better outcomes for patients who undergo repair of abdominal aortic aneurysms. It is felt that the patient has fewer post-op complications if the aorta is accessed through a lower oblique incision that is extended laterally so that the vessel is approached laterally or posteriorly rather than anteriorly. Organ transplant surgeries, such as kidney or liver transplants are most successful with this type of incision. This incision can also be lengthened to enable the surgery to have access to the inferior surface of the diaphragm and the vessels that intersect there.

Pfannenstiel Incision

The Pfannenstiel incision is a transverse incision made very low in the abdomen, just above the bikini line. The underlying fascia is then transected by using a medial, or vertical, incision. This is frequently used with surgeries that require access to the pelvic cavity, such as an abdominal hysterectomy or Cesarean section for delivery. By using both medial and transverse incisions, the wound tends to be very strong when it heals. Patients are usually pleased with the minimal scarring that is left because the transverse incision tends to follow a natural skin fold and is low enough that it cannot usually be seen while wearing normal clothes. The Pfannenstiel incision results in good exposure to the central pelvis but limits exposure to the lateral compartments of the pelvis and upper abdomen. It is not usually used for an abdominal surgery if it is suspected that multiple lymph node dissection will need to be performed due to cancer metastasis.

Use of Scalpels for Dissection

The scalpel can be fitted with various types of blades, described by number, depending on the purpose. For general surgical incisions, the #10 or #20 blades are frequently used because the blade is straight to prevent beveling of the incision edges. The scalpel is generally held between the thumb and middle fingers with the index finger either placed next to the middle finger or on top of the scalpel to apply pressure while making the surgical incision. When tissues need to be dissected, the scalpel is generally held like a pencil. This is necessary to perform exact movements. Smaller scalpel blades will be used for dissection to prevent unnecessary trauma to the surrounding tissues. Some blades are more curved than others and some are more elongated than others to come to a sharper point at the tip. There are other scalpel blades that are manufactured for specific surgeries or types of dissection.

The CRNFA is responsible for lightly stretching the skin and holding it firmly in place while the surgeon makes the surgical incision. This helps to provide upturned skin edges on the incision, decreasing the risk of poor wound healing because of down-turned wound edges. This also helps to keep the incision straight without multiple stops and starts. This prevents unnecessary lengthening of the incision. Patient safety is very important in the operating room, but the CRNFA must also be concerned with his or her own safety and the safety of the other members of the operating team. Always be conscious of the location of the scalpel to prevent injury and sudden movements that can cause inadvertent stab or cutting wound from the scalpel. Never try to pass the scalpel from person to person. It should be laid down on a sterile area of the operating team and then picked up by the person who needs to use it.

Surgical Scissors

Surgical scissors are available in multiple styles, but Metzenbaum scissors and Mayo scissors are the two that are used most often. The scissors vary in size, whether the tips of the scissors are sharp or dull, and whether the sharpened ends are straight or curved. Metzenbaum scissors are sharp and often used for dissection. By using a sharp tip, unnecessary trauma to the surrounding tissues is avoided that would be present with using blunt tips. The Metzenbaum scissors has an end that is slightly curved which makes them easier to manipulate. Mayo scissors are larger and heavier. They are most often used when cutting thick tissues. They also have an end that is slightly curved to facilitate maneuverability. There are other types of scissors that are made that vary in size and functional purpose. Some are manufactured for specific surgeries, including micro-surgeries, to provide better control for a specified procedure.

Dissection

First, the scissors must be held properly. The thumb should be placed through one ring and the ring finger though the other. The index and middle fingers will then provide support and improve control while handling the scissors. Once the area to be dissected is well-visualized with adequate lighting present, traction should be applied to the area to facilitate easy cutting and separation with the scissors. The tip of the scissors is inserted into the tissue only to the level at which the cut should be made. Repeated dissection may need to be performed to adequately expose an area. Of course, extreme care should be taken to prevent any damage to surrounding organs or tissue. Dissection with scissors should always be performed at an angle that follows the natural curve of the area being dissected. Forcing dissection in an angular plane from the area can result in unnecessary tissue damage.

Retractors

By the late 1800s, there was some understanding of the effects of excessive tissue handling and damage during surgery in relation to infection and poor patient outcomes. Dr. Halsted, an American surgeon, began perfecting a surgical technique that minimizes the amount of unnecessary tissue that occurred during surgery. He promoted clean incisions of tissue in the surgical site versus bluntly dissecting tissues. He also felt that the fewer internal sutures present at the surgical site, the less likely the patient would develop an infection. He believed that simple direct pressure to areas with a small amount of bleeding would result in hemostasis with excess suturing. He also educated other surgeons on using clamps effectively to prevent damage to surrounding healthy tissues. His work helped to lay the ground work toward lowering the infection rates following surgery, as well as providing the patient with better surgical outcomes through uncomplicated wound healing.

The hands are the ideal retractor to be used during surgery. Unnecessary pressure on tissues can usually be prevented because of the fine control that can be used when holding the tissues. The hands are also more flexible to help maintain anatomic position of the tissues or organs that are being retracted. Safety is a very big concern when using the hands for retractors. The CRNFA should ensure that the hands are not blocking any part of the surgical site. Awareness of the actions being performed in the surgical site should also be recognized to prevent accidental needle sticks or stab wounds with a scalpel. The hands can become easily fatigued during retraction, though, depending on the amount of force or pressure that is used. It is important to let the surgeon know if there is a risk of the retracted tissues slipping out of grasp to prevent any injury during surgery.

When surgery is performed in an area that requires tissues need to be retracted for a length of time longer than recommended when using regular retractors. Sutures are also useful in more delicate areas to separate critical structures be lifted out of the way to prevent injury or damage. Using sutures for retraction also provides a more gentle option for tissue retraction rather than using firm retractors in smaller, more critical areas of the body. Surgeries performed on the eye involve placing sutures through the tissue making up the eye lid and then gently retracting that tissue to hold it back to provide better visualization of the surgical site. The sutures may be held back by the CRNFA or attached to the towel or drape in the operating field using a clamp or hemostat. Sometimes a small piece of felt is placed between the suture material and the tissue that is being retracted. This prevents the fine suture from indenting on the tissue too severely which can lead to damage.

The retractors function to carefully and safely provide adequate exposure to the operative site by holding back tissues or organs that would otherwise be blocking the area. There are many types and styles of retractors and each type is indicated for a specific function or procedure. The CRNFA should be familiar with every type of retractor and how they are used. It is important to be very conscious of any unnecessary tissue damage that can occur by not using a retractor properly. Proper body mechanics should also be utilized when using retractors to prevent muscle soreness and fatigue. There are some retractors that do not require an extra person to be present in the operating room. Some of these open within the surgical site and then lock into place. Others are actually affixed to the operating room table and provide retraction that could otherwise require another person be present. Retractors that do not need to be repositioned while personnel take turns holding them can help to decrease the operating time.

Hand-Held Retractors

Many retractors have a handle at one end for the CRNFA to use for positioning the retractor. Holding retractors for prolonged periods of time can cause a good deal of fatigue, so the amount of pressure used during retraction may be adjusted at different phases of an operation. Care should be taken when placing the retractor. Prolonged pressure by the retractor on the surrounding tissues can decrease blood flow and lead to necrosis. If nerve fibers are present, compression on the nerves can cause motor or sensory deficits following surgery. When pulling the retractor toward you, the retractor should be gripped in the dominant hand in a fist and the tissues pulled gently toward you. When holding open a smaller incision away from the body, the retractor should be held like a pencil with gentle pressure applied to separate the wound edges. The surgeon's visibility should also be considered when holding retractors. Care should be taken to ensure his or her view is not blocked by the First Assistant.

Self-Retaining Retractors

Self-retaining retractors function to provide adequate retraction for the operative site to be visible, with an added bonus of utilizing the First Assistant to assist in surgery rather than just hold retractors in place. This is especially helpful in more complex surgeries where the extra hands of the CRNFA are necessary to the surgeon. Self-retaining retractors are frequently used in open chest surgeries to provide retraction of the sternum and rib cage. There are certain types of retractors that may be used for large abdominal surgeries.

Before placing the retractor, the tissues are examined for any structures that could potentially be damaged by retraction. The retractor is placed within the operative site and very slowly opened to ensure the blades are where they should be. Sponges may be placed between the tissues and the blades to provide cushioning. The tissues should be regularly checked during surgery for any damage or interruption in blood flow.

Allis Clamp

The Allis clamp is designed to be used on fragile tissues, such as organs. It comes in a variety of sizes and is classified by the size and quantity of the teeth located on its clamping ends. Because the clamps have teeth, it can exert a good deal of pressure with very little force. This provides the CRNFA a means by which to assist in retracting tissue without incurring excessive arm and hand fatigue. Allis clamps have also been used when placing internal sutures during surgery. Because they grasp tissue well but are designed for more delicate tissue, they can be used to maneuver tissue and portions of organs to further inspect an area. If bleeding has occurred, they can be used to manually remove clotted blood from the area. A drawback to using Allis clamps for retraction, as with any instruments, is that they may impair the surgeon's view of the operative site.

Kocher Instrument

The Kocher instrument is used for retracting very heavy tissue that may contain a significant amount of scar tissue. This helps to prevent the CRNFA from manually retracting this tissue, which can cause excessive hand and arm fatigue. The Kocher is effective at clamping this dense tissue because it exerts a great deal of pressure to the tissue. Scar tissue is very fibrous and can be difficult to retract from the surgical site, which can impair the surgeon's ability to adequately visualize the surgical field. Kocher instruments are also used when a patient has a midline incision for abdominal surgery. The Kocher clamp is used for holding onto the thick, dense fascia tissue to keep the edges well-approximated while sutures are being placed. As the CRNFA moves down the fascia, placing sutures, the clamp is removed and used to grasp the fascia further down to aid in pulling more tissue together for sutures.

Tenaculum

A tenaculum is similar to an Allis clamp in that there are teeth lining the clamping ends of the instrument, however, it tends to exert more force and is used on stronger tissue than the Allis clamp. Because of this, the tenaculum is most often used for lifting and moving more dense tissue while avoiding overexertion of pressure on it which could cause damage. The tenaculum is frequently used for grasping the cervix, especially during biopsy procedures. It has been found that this may cause pain and a topical anesthetic is frequently used before grasping the tissue. This may be reapplied to prevent an increase in pain if the tenaculum is used repeatedly or for an extended period of time. The tenaculum is also used in some vascular surgeries to grasp vessels that will be severed and tied. Because the clamps are lined with teeth, there is decreased surface area grasping tissue which can result in less tissue damage.

Babcock Clamp

While Kocher and Allis clamps exert a great deal of pressure on the tissue to provide firm retraction, the Babcock clamp is used in a more delicate manner for gentle lifting and moving of tissues. It is especially useful to lift intestinal tissue, the appendix, and any other tubular structures. The Babcock clamp does not have teeth along its clamping end, so it does not actually clamp down firmly on tissue. This greatly reduces the risk of significant tissue damage. The handle of the clamp does have a ratchet to fix the clamp in position, but it is not tightened enough to exert force on the tissue. Rather, it should be closed just enough to hold the tissue without firmly compressing it. One of the difficulties of using a Babcock clamp is that it does not provide a firm grip on tissues. If it is not ratcheted tightly enough, the bowel or other tissue may slip out which could obstruct the operative site

Choosing the Appropriate Retractor

The first factor to consider when choosing a retractor is the type of surgery to be performed. Large abdominal surgeries will require a significant amount of exposure for the surgeon and a large retractor may be necessary. Smaller surgeries with a smaller incision will require a smaller retractor. The structures to be retracted should be considered. More delicate vascular areas or tissues containing nerves will need to be more delicately retracted than other, more resilient tissues. Another factor to consider is the amount of force that will be necessary to hold the retractor in place. If several large structures are being retracted, more force will be required. The length of the operation will be a factor. Extended retraction will require a retractor that is comfortable to hold in place, or possibly a self-retaining retractor. Patient size should also be considered when choosing a retractor. Patients with a large body girth will have more fatty tissue that will need to be held back to provide adequate visualization of the surgical site.

Sponges

Sponges can function to absorb blood and fluid or to help with organ retraction. If bleeding within the surgical site is slow, sponges can be moistened with sterile saline and placed at the site of bleeding They should be allowed to absorb the blood until they are either over saturated or until the bleeding stops. Sponges may help with hemostasis when held over an area that is bleeding with some pressure applied. Sponges can facilitate visualization into an area for surgery. An organ can be carefully moved to the side using the hand and a sponge placed under the edge of the organ and tucked into the incision flap. This will protect the organ and provide some retraction for surgery. To prevent retractors from causing unnecessary tissue damage, sponges can be placed between the blade of the retractor and the tissue being retracted and serve as a cushion. It is important that a careful sponge count is maintained during surgery to prevent a sponge accidentally being left in the patient.

CRNFA Assistance During Suturing

The CRNFA should know ahead of time what time of suturing material is appropriate for different types of surgical wounds. He or she should also know what the surgeon prefers. This material should be ready for use when it is time to close the incision. The surgeon may prefer the CRNFA close the incision, he or she may prefer to do it on their own, or the suturing may be a team effort. If the CRNFA is assisting the surgeon with closure, assistance may be given with providing traction on the skin to assist with exposing the needle after the bite is made. The CRNFA may also tie knots on the tail end of the suture as the surgeon creates additional stitches in the incision. Once the stitches are created and the knots are tied, the CRNFA may also help by holding the tails with some counter force so that the excess suture line can be cut.

Eyes of Suture Needles

The eye of the suture needle is the location where the suture material is attached to the needle. There are three different types. The closed-eye needle has a hole that is threaded with the suture material, similar to a regular sewing needle. The edges of the eye are very smooth to prevent fraying of the suture material. This type of needle can be sterilized and reused. The French-eye (split-eye) needle has a spring mechanism that allows for easier threading of the suture material. They are not commonly used because needles with this type of eye are generally very small and only used in very specialized surgeries. Swaged (atraumatic) needles do not have an eye and the suture material is attached to the end of the needle without any break in the contour of the needle. This is the most common type of suture needle used and is disposable. There is a type that allows the needle to be broken off to prevent accidental needle sticks when suturing is completed.

Needle Shapes

Suturing needles with a slight curve, such as one-quarter circle needles and compound curved needles, are primarily used in eye surgeries. The one-quarter circle needle may also be used in microscopic surgeries. The one-half circle and five-eighths circle needles are more curved and require more manipulation of the wrist to properly "bite" the tissue when creating sutures. These are useful, though when in a deep, crowded space because of the ability to completely visualize the tip after initially inserting the needle into the tissue that is to be sutured. The most commonly used suture needle is the three-eighths circle needle. It provides a slight curvature, but is comfortable for creating sutures and is commonly used for basic skin lacerations and surgical closure of the skin. The straight needle is rarely used because of its decreased flexibility and limited use, along with an increased risk of needle stick injury associated with it.

Shaft of the Suture Needle

The shaft, or body, of the needle is the main section of the suturing needle between the eye and the point. It can vary in width and even in shape. It may also be straight or curved depending on its use. Some needles can vary in shape, for example, there may be an indented area of the body of the needle in the area where it would be gripped for suturing. Curved needles can vary from forming a quarter of a circle up to curving into over one-half of a circle. The degree of curvature will affect the degree of difficulty the CRNFA will have in creating the sutures. The more curved the needle is, the more dexterity is necessary to manipulate the needle when placing the sutures. Straight needles are not used as frequently as curved needles because of the increased risk of accidental needle stick when using them. There is also not a lot of maneuverability with a straight needle.

Points on Suture Needles

Suturing needles can have points that are sharp, or cutting, tapered, or blunt. The cutting needles have a triangular-shaped body and are very sharp. They are frequently used for penetrating thicker tissues, including connective tissue and some bone. Sutures can be placed in tendons using this type of suturing needle. The tapered-point suturing needles have a round body. They are used throughout the GI tract as well as for suturing muscle and fat tissue. Surgeries performed in the oropharyngeal cavity may include sutures using this type of suturing needle. The blunt-point needles have a round body, also. They have been used more frequently to prevent the risk of needle stick that can occur with the sharp suturing needles. It is used primarily for organs of the gastrointestinal tract as well as in connective tissue. There has been some concern that blunt needles may cause some minor tissue trauma when used.

Needle Holders

Needle holders are used for exactly what their name says, to hold the needle while suturing an incision. They are available in different sizes and weights. The important part of selecting an appropriate needle holder for suturing is to ensure it is in the correct size and will not damage the needle. Needle holders are usually blunt tipped and have ringed hands and the ability to ratchet closed. The needle is grasped just distal to the eye of the needle. The needle should be positioned within the needle holder so that the curvature of the needle is perpendicular to the straight edge of the instrument. Once positioned correctly in the needle holder, the handles are ratcheted to secure the needle in place. Holding the needle holder, the needle is directed through the patient's skin at about a 90-degree angle and the needle holder is rotated to drive the needle back out through the skin. The exact technique for placing sutures using needle holders will vary depending on the type of suture to be used.

Grips to Hold Needle Holders During Suturing

The palmed grip is used when the needle is driven through very thick tissue. The needle holder is held in the palm of the hand and gripped in the fist so that a lot of strength can be used to drive the needle through the tissue. The thenar grip is used to facilitate placing sutures quickly. The needle holder is held with the ring handle held against the thenar surface of the thumb. This helps to provide support on the needle holder while still maintaining control. The thumb-ring finger grip is used most often and involves placing the thumb and ring finger in the ring handles. This allows for easy repositioning of the needle and for opening and closing the ratchet closure easily. The pencil grip is only used for small needle holders used in very delicate surgeries. It has a latch closure that is controlled with pressure from the fingers. The needle may be difficult to control using this type of needle holder because of the fine control necessary to operate it correctly.

Forceps for Suturing

Forceps are used along with the needle holder and suture needle. They can be used to pull the tip of the suture through the skin once the point of the needle has broken through the skin surface. The needle is then held still with the forceps so that it can be secured with the needle holders. When the suture needle is driven through the tissue to approximate wound edges, the forceps can be used to apply pressure on the skin through which the needle will exit. This facilitates exit of the needle so the stitch can be completed. Forceps are available in many different styles, including tips that have teeth to assist with grasping tissue. If this type of forceps is used to assist with suturing, care should be taken to avoid any unnecessary tissue trauma that can occur from the teeth cutting into the tissue. Forceps of appropriate weight should be used to ensure they are capable of exerting enough pressure on the tissue without damaging the instrument.

Suture Scissors

Suture scissors are available in several different sizes. The blades may be angulated or may follow a straight line. Suture scissors are held the same way forceps are held with the thumb and fourth fingers in the handles. The index finger is used to stabilize the scissors. Scissors are primarily used to cut the "tails," or ends of the suture line that is remaining after a stitch is created. The amount of tail left at the knot depends upon the location and type of sutures created. Regular continuous or interrupted sutures used for surgical wound closure generally have about ¼-inch of tail left intact to facilitate easy grasping for suture removal. Suture scissors are also used for removing sutures once the surgical incision is healed. An incision is made just underneath the knot that the suture line is pull in a direction that will prevent the suture material that was on the skin surface from being pulled under the skin through the healed wound.

Blunt Needles vs. Sharp Needles

Approximately one-half of the stabbing injuries in the operating room occur because of needle sticks. These are usually due to the person doing the suturing sticking themselves, but the assistant, or CRNFA, can also be accidentally stuck with the suture needle. Suture needles with a blunt tip can greatly decrease the number of stick injuries that occur during surgery. Most surgeons who have used blunt-tipped needles have not felt that they are more difficult to use and they have not had problems with driving the needle through tissue. It is felt that any trauma that may occur to the tissue because of the extra force necessary to use the needle is very minimal. Blunt needles are now available in many different sizes and styles. Because of the positive results seen in studies that have been conducted, it has been suggested that blunt needles should be used whenever possible to prevent the increased risk of a penetrating injury in the operating room.

Knots Used in Suturing

The 3 main types of knots used when suturing are described below:

- The square knot is used most often and is very strong. It involves creating a simple knot and then repeating the simple knot, but looping the tail of the suture in the opposite direction. This results in a square appearance when the knot is examined.
- The surgeon's knot is used in areas when there is tissue tension in the area. It is created by tying two consecutive overhand, or simple, knots in a row without pulling the first one tight. After drawing the suture line tight, a simple knot is created.

- The granny knot is a slip knot that is secured by creating a square knot on top of it. The granny knot can be tightened and is most helpful in surgical sites that are very small and confined. This is often used on incisions that require internal absorbable sutures because of usually needing to place these sutures in an enclosed area.

Absorbable Sutures

Absorbable sutures can be manufactured using natural or man-made materials. They are designed to have decreased strength over a varying amount of time. Some types of absorbable sutures are treated with materials that facilitate this process even quicker.

The most common kind of absorbable suture used is catgut which is made from sheep tissue. It begins losing its strength within just a few hours of surgery. A form of man-made, or synthetic, absorbable suture is Vicryl which is very commonly used. It is broken down by enzymes in the body. The strength of synthetic sutures and the time it will take for them to completely break down will vary from brand to brand. The important issue to consider when using absorbable sutures is that a brand is chosen that will provide the strength needed to aid in wound healing for the amount of time they are necessary before they dissolve.

Absorbable sutures can be natural or synthetic and the different types have different uses. Natural sutures, or "gut", are usually used for more superficial soft tissue incisions and in eye surgeries. These are avoided in deeper cardiothoracic or neurovascular surgeries because of their rapid rate of absorption. Because natural absorbable sutures are protein-based, they can fray when used and may not have the strength that synthetic absorbable sutures can provide. Natural absorbable sutures should also not be used in patients who are allergic to collagen substances because there can be cross-reactivity. The synthetic absorbable sutures are also used for soft tissue suturing. Like all absorbable sutures, they should not be used for suturing tissue that performs stressed motions. This includes cardiovascular structures. There is one type of synthetic monofilament suture material that is indicated for use in pediatric cardiovascular surgeries. Generally, the synthetic absorbable sutures will require more time, up to over 200 days, to completely absorb compared to natural absorbable suture material.

Nonabsorbable Sutures

Nonabsorbable sutures can be made from silk or cotton or can be man-made. They maintain their strength for a much greater time than the absorbable sutures. Nonabsorbable sutures are frequently used internally to provide reconnection, or anastomosis, of bowel following resection and these sutures are left intact. Other forms of nonabsorbable surgical incision closure include glue (Dermabond) and staples. Skin glue is used for incisions that are not on an area that is subject to flexing stress, and is especially useful for cosmetic purposes with facial surgeries. Surgical staples are very quick to use and generally provide good strength for wound closure to facilitate healing. These are generally used in areas that need extra support to hold a surgical incision closed, such as some abdominal incisions and long incisions created for orthopedic surgeries. Some surgical incisions may be closed using both absorbable and nonabsorbable sutures. The absorbable sutures are used to close underlying tissues while nonabsorbable sutures or staples are used to close the superficial tissues.

Nonabsorbable sutures are generally sturdier and have more uses than absorbable sutures. They are made from different materials, including silk, nylon, and even steel. Silk nonabsorbable sutures are generally used for soft tissue incisions including cardiothoracic and neurovascular surgeries. In some individuals, an autoimmune rejection reaction can occur with silk sutures. Nylon sutures can be monofilament or braided. They are also used for general soft tissue closure including cardiovascular and neurological procedures. They can also be used for closure in eye surgeries. Patients are unlikely to suffer an allergic reaction to these. Steel nonabsorbable sutures are used for closure of large structures, such as sternum repair following open chest surgery. Patients are unlikely to have an allergic reaction to this material, but those with nickel allergies should not receive steel sutures. There is a risk that the steel suture material can break if there is excessive bending or twisting of the suture.

Continuous Sutures

Continuous sutures are faster to create and provide one line of sutures without multiple knots. The needle is driven through both edges of the wound at one end. A knot is tied and then the needle is driven through the opposing edges down the entire length of the incision. Once the end of the incision is reached, another knot is tied to secure the line of sutures in place. The problem is that the tension can vary throughout the line of sutures which can cause a puckering effect at one end of the incision. The tension of the suture must remain the same throughout the line of sutures to promote proper wound healing and prevent cosmetic problems with the wound. Care should also be taken to prevent the wound edges from become misaligned. Overall, there is a more obvious scar present with continuous sutures than with interrupted sutures. The location of the incision should be considered when using continuous sutures because of the possibility of a residual scar.

Following a Suture

The CRNFA can help the surgeon while continuous sutures are placed by following the suture. This prevents excessive tension from being applied to the suture line and helps to facilitate an evenly closed incision with wound edges that are well-approximated. As the surgeon places a suture, the suture line is held with forceps while the surgeon begins the next stitch. The suture material can be held with the fingers also, but this will not be possible when the suture line becomes too short. Also, the fingers can be too large and can interfere with the surgeon's ability to see the tissue clearly in order to place the next suture in the correct place. Following a suture is very effective, but can be a learned skill. The surgeon and CRNFA need to work closely together to ensure the suture is not released too early and that the appropriate amount of tension is placed on the line to prevent gapping of the wound or puckering of the wound when drawn too tight.

Interrupted Sutures

Interrupted sutures are individual sutures that are placed to approximate wound edges. They are favored over continuous sutures in areas of the body that may experience more stress. The extra support of an individual knot at each suture helps to provided added strength and prevent gaping of the wound edges. Interrupted sutures take longer to create because of the process of placing each suture individually with tying the knot and cutting the suture after each knot. Individual sutures have the advantage of maintaining accurate approximation of the wound edges. The risk of misalignment and uneven tension placed on the wound edges is decreased because of placing sutures individually instead of pulling the tissue with continuous sutures. When interrupted sutures are removed, there is less risk of pulling suture material that may be covered with bacteria, due to being on the external surface of the skin, through the wound bed itself.

Subcutaneous Sutures

Subcutaneous sutures are not always used when closing a surgical incision. They may be necessary, though, in wounds that are very deep with a significant amount of subcutaneous overlying them. They are also used to prevent dead space within the wound so that proper healing can occur. When creating subcutaneous sutures, care should be taken to prevent excessive tension on the tissue which can interfere with its blood supply. The sutures are also placed very close together which helps to avoid any spaces in the subcutaneous tissue. Absorbable suture material is usually used to avoid leaving suture line in the wound for an excessive period of time. When creating subcutaneous sutures, avoid taking too deep of a "bite" in the tissue because of the potential for organ or blood vessel damage underneath. This can occur if the suture needle pierces an organ or vessel. Once subcutaneous sutures are placed, the superficial tissue and skin can be sutured to provide complete closure of the incision.

Interrupted Mattress Sutures

Interrupted mattress sutures are used in incisions that are in an area of the body that may receive a lot of tension. They provide more reinforcement and a stronger closure than regular interrupted sutures. Mattress sutures are created by driving the suture needle through the skin and out within the wound. A second "bite" is made as the needle is then driven from within the wound and out through the skin on the other side of the incision. Mattress sutures can also be created by inserting the suture needle at a distance farther than normal from the incision. This produces an overall longer stitch which provides more stability since more tissue is involved. Like all sutures, when removing interrupted mattress sutures, be sure to cut the suture line close to the skin and pull in the direction that prevents the exposed suture material from being dragged through the incision itself.

Skin Staples

Skin staples are small staples that are placed, using forceps, to hold a wound closed for healing. They are very easy to use and leave a less noticeable scar than with most sutures.

A special device is used to insert the staples. Both edges of the surgical incision are approximated to each other with the edges slightly everted. The staple is then placed using the device, similar to a staple gun. This requires two people while one will hold one edge of the incision with forceps and the other can hold the opposing edge of the incision and operate the stapler. Skin staples are very similar to regular staples in that they are driven straight into the skin and tissue below and then the edges are bent to hold them in place. When the sutures are ready to be removed, a special staple removal is used that will crimp the back of the staple and cause the bent edges to straighten so the staple can be gently pulled out.

Dressings for Nondraining Wounds

The primary purpose of the surgical incision dressing is to protect the healing wound from becoming infected while promoting adequate healing at the site. This is accomplished by providing a semipermeable dressing that allows air and water to enter the area, and keeps the area moist to promote cell growth. A draining wound would require a dressing that prevents the drainage from contacting surrounding healthy skin to prevent breakdown of that skin. The surgical incision site should be clean before a dressing is applied. Once this is accomplished, a clean dressing is applied and secured into place using type or self-adhesive. This should be non-irritating to the surrounding skin. The process of changing the surgical incision dressing should not be too complicated so that it can be easily taught to the patient before discharge home. If the wound requires packing or other special care, home health may need to become involved to perform wound dressing changes at home.

Surgical Drains

Drains are used when there is residual bleeding internally at a surgical site or when there is an infection present that is draining purulent material. The tubing connected to the drain has its tip at the site of drainage and it is passed through the body wall to connect to the drain or other form of suction. The drain tubing should not pass through the original surgical incision site, but an opening should be made away from the site. This helps to reduce the risk of infection at the surgical site. The drainage tubing is secured in place at the skin to prevent slipping of the tubing or retraction of the tubing into the surgical site. Drains can serve as sites of infection with the opening through the body wall and the tubing serving as a means by which bacteria can enter the surgical site. It is important to leave a drain in place for as minimal amount of time as possible to prevent possible complication from infection.

Forceps

Forceps are used for grasping and picking up objects. They are held in the hand like a pencil and are very helpful and easy to use once you become comfortable with the feel of them in your hand. There are several different styles of forceps. The length can vary, as well as the width. The tips can be smooth or have a series of teeth that provide a better grip for grasping. Forceps without teeth are generally used on more delicate tissues, while forceps with teeth are used on more sturdy tissues that are not as easily susceptible to damage. Care should always be taken to avoid grasping tissue too firmly because of the risk of tissue damage. Grasping too firmly can also cause the forceps to slip off the tissue which can lead to tissue injury. Tissues should be held with the forceps for as short a period as possible to avoid damage from excessive compression.

THUMB FORCEPS

There are several different types of thumb forceps available and they have many different uses to help with manipulating tissue during surgery. They are available with a smooth tip or a tip with teeth for stronger grasping capabilities. There are also different types of thumb forceps which are specially designed for a specific procedure. The tips of the thumb forceps extend from the thumb and from the ends of the other fingers. This tends to give an effect as if the thumb and fingers were extended, which can help with fine grasping skills. They are easiest to use when held like a pencil. Thumb forceps are used for grasping tissue that needs to be lifted or removed. They are valuable when used in conjunction with a needle holder while suturing. Thumb forceps are also used to grasp the needle while suturing and a longer version can be used to pack and remove sponges in the operative site.

CLAMPS

Clamps are also used to grasp tissue and sponges, but they vary from forceps in that they have a scissors-type handle and the ability to lock into place while grasping tissue. Clamps will vary in size and weight. The tips can also vary from smooth to those with teeth. Some clamps have tips that are curved and there are clamps that are designed to be used in specific surgeries. Multiple clamps may be used at the same time to simultaneously grasp tissue that needs to be retracted. When the clamps are in use, it is advisable that they be held on the shaft rather than through the finger hooks. This helps to prevent the lock from being jarred and possibly released prematurely during surgery. Like forceps, clamped tissue needs to be regularly assessed for any damage or decrease in blood flow to the area. Tissue should be release as soon as possible to prevent excessive compression and resultant damage.

HEMOSTATS

The CRNFA is responsible for providing a clear surgical field without obstructions that may prevent the surgeon from performing the surgery. When a vessel, whether small or large, is severed, bleeding can be profuse enough to interfere with the surgery. It is the responsibility of the CRNFA to control this bleeding quickly to facilitate a smooth surgery. Hemostats can be used to control bleeding and are available in many different styles. There are types that provided a textured, or serrated, surface on the clamps which can improve grip. Hemostats are used to clamp a vessel and stop bleeding. The vessel is clamped while preventing the least amount of trauma possible. If a vessel is going to be severed, two hemostats are clamped onto the vessel and the vessel is cut between the two instruments. If a branch off a main vessel is to be clamped, the hemostat should be placed a short distance away from the main vessel to prevent damage to that vessel.

Handling Techniques

The CRNFA will need to use hemostats frequently so it is important to become very comfortable with using this instrument. As comfort increases, using the hemostats will not feel awkward and will come quite naturally. To clamp a bleeding vessel, the tips of the hemostat will be used. This allows compression to be placed on the end of the vessel to stop the bleeding, without causing extensive tissue damage with a serrated clamp. The vessel is secured in the hemostat from the end with the instrument coming off the vessel in a straight line. If the entire clamp, not just the tip, is used to compress a vessel, the hemostats are placed at a 90-degree angle from the vessel. When sutures are being placed, the hemostats should be held by the handles without using the finger rings. This facilitates easy movement of the instrument back and forth. The clamp of the hemostat is then slowly released as he sutures are completed.

Preventing Hemostat Burns

The lowest power setting possible should be used initially. If this is not effective, it can be adjusted later. But initially, always begin with the lowest setting. The hemostat operates with a monopolar charge so that a dispersing pad is placed somewhere on the patient to receive the charge through a return electrode. If the CRNFA cleans on the patient, there is the potential for that electric current to pass through him or her, which can lead to a shock occurring. Always have a firm grip on the hemostat without applying too much pressure which can lead to fatigue. A firm grasp on the instrument will prevent accidentally dropping the instrument when it is activated, which could lead to burning of healthy tissue accidentally. Always avoid applying the charged end of the hemostat to a metal object. This will cause sparking and may result in injury. Surgical gloves will not protect against any type of electric current injury.

Suctioning

Suctioning is used to remove blood and other body fluids from the operative site. Suction tools come in various shapes and sizes and will vary depending on the type of surgery being performed and the amount of blood loss expected during the surgery. Suctioning should be performed very carefully to avoid any trauma to the tissues within the area. Most suction devices have an opening on the shaft portion of the tool that is covered with the finger to increase the amount of suction provided. To avoid tissue damage while suctioning, suction should not be applied at full force directly against organ tissue. If organ tissue is absorbed into the suction tip, the suction should be discontinued and then the device removed from the area. Never force the suction tip off tissue while the suction is being applied because this can result in significant tissue trauma. Some suction devices may have small, removable parts that should be monitored during surgery to prevent them being "lost" in the operative site.

Closing Traumatic Wounds

The main concern with traumatic wounds is that of infection. Wounds that occurred many hours previously are much more likely to be infected with bacterial organisms. Closing this wound will trap those bacteria inside leading to infection and abscess formation. Generally, if a wound has been open for 6-8 hours, it is best to leave it open for healing by secondary intention. If the wound can be debrided and sufficiently cleaned, this time frame may be stretched some. The shape of the wound and the amount of surrounding tissue damage should also be considered. Jagged, ripped wounds are much more difficult to close than clean cut edges. Debridement may need to be performed to provide a clean closure to the wound. If there is massive tissue damage, there may not be enough surrounding skin and tissue to provide ample wound closure. Any surrounding tissue that has lost its blood supply should be debrided before wound closure can occur.

Primary Intention Wound Healing

Wounds can heal by primary intention if they are caused by a clean cut. This would include a surgical incision or a traumatic cut made by a knife or piece of glass. They are generally not dirty wounds, or caused by trauma, can be cleaned adequately using irrigation with sterile saline. This type of wound has edges that can be well-approximated with slightly everted edges and closed using skin glue, sutures, or surgical staples. There are generally no gaps in the incision line while healing occurs because the incision is a clean cut and the edges will draw together evenly. This type of wound usually heals without any complications, though infection can occur. This is more likely with traumatic wounds that may have a very small foreign body or bacteria trapped inside. Copious irrigation with sterile saline is essential to ensure the wound is as clean as possible before the edges are pulled together and sealed.

Secondary Intention Wound Healing

Wounds that heal by secondary intention are characterized by excessive tissue loss that prevents the use of sutures or staples for wound closure. These wounds are wide and left open to heal. If kept clean and moist, granulation tissue will form along the bottom of the wound and gradually fill in. This will be followed for the formation of scar tissue over the superficial surface of the wound, though the scar will be wide and not as cosmetically pleasing as the scar that is left behind after a wound that has healed by primary intention.

Tissue that has undergone excessive debridement may be left open to heal by secondary intention. This is necessary in a situation where an infection is present to avoid trapping bacteria within the wound. Traumatic wounds may also be left open to heal by secondary intention because there may be loss of tissue that prevents the wound edges from being well-approximated for suturing or stapling.

Tertiary Intention Wound Healing

Tertiary wound healing is similar to healing by secondary intention, except that the wound edges will be pulled together and sealed using sutures or staples after several days of healing. As the wound begins to heal and granulation tissue forms in the wound bed, the wound edges tend to draw slightly together. If enough of this contraction of the wound edges occurs, they can be pulled together to close the wound. The advantage of tertiary wound healing is the prevention of infection. The wound will not be left open for an excessive period of time, which decreases the chance of bacteria growing within it, leading to a wound infection. There can be more scarring with wound healing using the tertiary method, but cannot be avoided at times if the wound is very wide with excessive tissue loss. This most frequently occurs with traumatic wounds or wounds that are widened due to removal of tissue from debridement.

Phases of Wound Healing

Open Wounds

The healing process that occurs with an open wound is similar to that of a closed wound, except it may take longer for the proliferative phase to occur. Once the inflammatory process has completed, the inflammatory cells leave the area. They are replaced by cells that promote tissue growth and the development of granulation tissue within the wound bed. After just a few days, the wound edges begin to contract and continue doing so for approximately 2 weeks. At this point, the wound can be left to heal by secondary intention or, if possible, the wound edges may be drawn together and secured with sutures or staples which would be considered tertiary intention. Once the granulation tissue has filled the wound, the wound will body will lay down collagen over the area of new tissue to help increase strength and begin scar formation. This final phase can continue for several months.

Closed Wounds

There are three main phases to closed wound healing:

- The inflammatory phase begins within seconds of wound formation. This is the process by which platelets and clotting proteins form a clot at the wound site. Immune cells travel to the area and begin releasing substances that will destroy bacteria and dead tissue cells.
- The proliferative phase begins a few days after the wound is created and lasts for about 3 weeks. This is the stage at which healing is evident with scab tissue being replaced by soft skin and connective tissue. The wound edges close during this phase and protein is used to form collagen and create a strong base for the wound to enter its final phase of healing.
- The maturation phase occurs for months and is the stage in which the wound forms a scar and gains added strength. Once complete, the wound has reached its maximum strength.

Secondary Healing Wounds

A secondary healing wound is a wound that is beginning to heal that is then re-opened. Surprisingly, this type of wound will actually heal quicker than a wound healed by primary intention. There does not appear to be any delay in the wound healing process when this occurs. The end result after healing is completed is a more cosmetically pleasing scar with less scar tissue deposition. This type of wound occurs following wound dehiscence after surgery or when a traumatic wound is re-opened after the initial healing process has begun or after it has been sutured or stapled closed. It can also occur with wounds that are healing by secondary intention. Trauma can occur to granulation tissue that has formed. A secondary healing wound will become a healed wound that is just as strong as a wound that healed by primary intention without any complications during the healing process.

Preoperative Factors Contributing to Wound Healing

A patient's risk factors should be identified and addressed before surgery to prevent any complications of wound healing. Consideration should be given for appropriate administration of prophylactic antibiotics prior to surgery. It is recommended that antibiotics be given parenterally (IV) no longer than 2 hours before surgery begins. Most patients only need one dose of antibiotics, but patients undergoing more complicated surgeries may require more than one dose of antibiotics. Another factor to consider preoperatively is the length of time that the patient has had an open wound. If this is a traumatic injury and several hours have passed since the time of injury, it may be necessary for the patient to undergo extensive debridement and irrigation for proper removal of contaminated tissue. It may even be advisable to let the wound heal by secondary intention to prevent closure of a wound that could possibly be contaminated with bacteria. This would depend on the nature of the injury.

Interventions to Prevent Wound Complications

The wound should be carefully inspected regularly with its appearance documented in the patient's chart to record any change. Assess for any erythema, edema, warmth, or discharge. Note whether the wound edges are well-approximated or if there is gapping present. Also describe the patient's pain level using a 0 to 10 pain scale. If infection is suspected, document the characteristics of the wound discharge and measure the area of erythema or induration surrounding the wound. Also record the patient's vital signs to evaluate for an elevation in temperature. Patient education regarding wound dressing changes is important to ensure continuity of proper wound care at home. Verify that the patient or friend/family member that will be caring for the patient understand how to properly change the dressing and cleanse the wound. Also educate them on the signs and symptoms of infection along with name and phone number of the person to call if an infection is suspected.

Surgical Wound Types

Clean wounds are uncomplicated wounds that are usually not caused by any type of injury or trauma. This involves the skin and soft tissue without any organ involvement. An example of this would be a surgical incision for a soft tissue procedure. A clean-contaminated wound occurs when there is organ system involvement with the wound, but it is well-controlled. An example of this would be a colon resection surgery that is uncomplicated. A contaminated wound is usually caused by trauma. It involves the presence of some type of contaminant material into the wound itself. A dirty or infected wound is traumatic and similar to a contaminated wound, but this is the point at which an infection has occurred in the wound. It may even involve the perforation of an organ. This type of wound will require surgical repair with debridement of dead tissue and excessive irrigation for cleaning. Antibiotic therapy may also be required.

Risk Factors for Developing Wound Infections

Certain patients will have an increased risk for developing wound infections. Overall poor health and co-morbidities may place them at increased risk. For example, diabetes may impede wound healing and place the patient at risk for wound infection. Patients with vascular disease may not have adequate circulation to promote drainage of infectious materials or formation of an appropriate inflammatory reaction necessary for healing. A patient's nutritional status before surgery can impede their ability to fight infection and prevent wound complications. Patients receiving immunosuppressant therapies are also at risk for having an incompetent immune system that is not able to properly ward off infection. The risk of nosocomial, or hospital-acquired, infections increases with the length of hospital stay. If a prolonged hospitalization has been necessary, there is a higher risk of developing a wound infection. Patients who have been hospitalized for an extended period of time may also have had several invasive procedures along with IVs and catheters in place. This can provide a source of infection in the patient.

Abscess

An abscess is a localized, encapsulated infection. An infection develops at a wound and borders are formed around the central portion of infection. This is formed by bacteria and blood cells to wall off the infection into a capsule. The patient will develop a palpable, inflamed mass that is tender. A fever may or may not be present, as well as an elevated white blood cell count. Treatment of an abscess involves incising and draining the abscess and leaving the wound open to drain. This will prevent the re-formation of an abscess in the same location. If it is not treated, the abscess can leak bacterial material into the system and cause sepsis in the patient. Antibiotics may be given if a systemic infection is confirmed on blood cultures or if the abscess has extensive tissue damage and there is risk of re-infection or superimposed infection following incision and drainage of the abscess.

Wound Dehiscence

Wound dehiscence is an opening of the surgical incision. This usually occurs about 1 week after surgery and a serosanguinous discharge is usually present before the wound opens. If a wound becomes dehisced within the first few hours following surgery, it is usually resutured. Nonabsorbable sutures should be used because they provide extra strength to hold the wound closed. If dehiscence occurs after that time, it is usually packed and allowed to heal by secondary or tertiary intention. Tissue debridement may need to be performed as the wound heals. As the wound heals, a ridge will develop along the incision line as collagen and connective tissue cells are deposited. Wounds that do not develop this ridge are more likely to dehisce because of a lack of tensile strength. This is considered a serious complication of surgery and can have a mortality rate up to 30% following some procedures. Fortunately, wound dehiscence occurs in only approximately 2% of surgeries performed.

Causes of Nonhealing Wounds

There are multiple forms of cancer that result in nonhealing wounds. These include the lesions commonly seen with basal cell, squamous cell, and malignant melanoma. Leukemia can also cause ulcerative wounds that will have delayed healing. There are situations in which a patient sustains repeated trauma to an area, such as with poor personal care habits that lead to continued skin infections from bacterial invasion. Patients may also have chronic skin infections that can cause pruritus which may lead to wounds that remain chronic and will not heal. Chronic vascular disease, arterial or venous, can lead to skin ulcers that will be nonhealing. When blood circulation is compromised, the adequate nutrition and immune factors cannot be present in the area to promote wound healing and tissue growth. The risk for vascular disease is increased in patients with diabetes. Patients who undergo radiation treatments for treatment of cancer can develop dermatitis and damage to the skin. Skin breakdown can occur which may result in wounds that have prolonged healing.

Seromas and Hematomas

A seroma is a collection of blood and immune cells located underneath the surgical incision. It can result from bleeding disorders, increased movement following surgery, or, most likely, from a bleeding vessel within the wound. A seroma contains a clear-yellowish thin fluid while a hematoma contains blood. Depending upon their location, they can compress vital organs or structures around them with can lead to complications. Though these fluid collections are not considered infections of the wound, they can lead to an infection. To prevent this complication, the fluid should be aspirated using aseptic technique. In severe cases, the surgical incision may need to be reopened and drained. If a bleeding vessel is the cause of the hematoma, ligation may need to be performed to control the bleeding. Seromas frequently develop near the surgical incision following mastectomy surgery. This is particularly true if lymph nodes and vessels in the area are removed, which help to facilitate drainage of fluid.

Epithelial Cyst

An epithelial cyst usually occurs when sutures are left in place too long. As part of the healing process, epithelial cells travel to the area where the sutures are placed in the skin. They will line the area around the suture material, but if the suture is in place too long, an excessive number of epithelial cells can congregate in one location which will form a cyst. Epithelial cysts can also occur in non-surgical patients because of an excessive accumulation of epidermal cells in one area. These are usually flesh colored, though some may have a darker colored center. Whether due to a surgical incision or if they occur in a patient who has not had surgery, epithelial cysts are usually left untreated. If they occur in an area that compromises vision or function, they can be surgically removed and covered by insurance. Insurance will not provide payment for removal of an epithelial cyst for cosmetic reasons.

Incisional Hernia

A hernia is a weakening in the wall of fascia that results in a protrusion of bowel through the opening. An incisional hernia occurs when there is a weakening in the tissue that makes up the incision, allowing protrusion of the underlying tissue. Incisional hernias occur after the wound has healed. An infection can cause a permanent weakening of the tissue around the incision, which can lead to weakening of that area after the healing process has completed. Improper technique with wound closure can also contribute to the development of an incisional hernia. If sutures are not placed properly, the tissue edges may not be well-approximated and the wound may not have adequate tensile strength. Obese patients with an obtunded abdomen have increased stress applied to the abdominal wall which can cause an increased load against the incision. This can contribute to the weakening that results in an incisional hernia.

Hypertrophic Scars and Keloids

Hypertrophic, or keloid, scars have a predilection for forming in certain populations, especially African-American patients. As a surgical incision or traumatic wound is healing, the body responds by depositing excessive collagen tissue. This results in a large, growth-like mass at the incision site. Keloids can appear as overgrown flesh-colored lesions along the scar. There may be some normal scar formation at an incision along with keloid tissue. Patients who are known keloid-formers may be given steroids during the wound healing phase to suppress the body's natural tendency to form keloids. There has been some success with direct injection of steroids at the incision site, also. Some patients have opted to have the keloids surgically removed, but there is a risk of forming another keloid at the surgery site. There has been success with removing the keloids using cryotherapy, or freezing. Laser therapy can also be effective at decreasing the size of keloid scars.

Suture Sinuses and Sinus Tracts

A sinus tract can occur due to the sutures themselves or because of an infection. A sinus is defined as an opening, or tunneling, through the skin. A sinus is present when sutures are removed, but these will heal spontaneously when the suture tracts are filled with skin cells. When an abscess occurs due to infection, a sinus tract can form that is a tunneling of infectious material. A cotton-tipped applicator can often be carefully pushed through the sinus to fully assess the depth of the sinus. Most sinus tracts due to infection will heal after antibiotic treatment and/or incision and drainage of the abscess occurs. In some cases, the sinus tracts may be extensive enough that they will need to be opened and irrigated. These will often be left open to heal by secondary intention. Tertiary healing can also be used in sinus tract healing by allowing some granulation tissue to form in the sinus after the infectious is removed and then suturing or stapling the incision closed.

Types of Wound Pain

There are two types of wound pain. Acute wound pain is present in the immediate post-operative period and is responsive to analgesic medications. It is usually temporary and begins to diminish a few days following surgery, depending on the type of procedure that was performed. Late post-operative wound pain can be chronic and occurs after the surgical incision has healed. This can be due to late development of an infection within the wound, a rare complication of a device or sponge retained in the surgical site, chronic pain following bone fusion or prosthesis placement, or neurologic pain. Neurologic pain following surgery can resolve with time or may be chronic. It is not unusual for superficial nerve fibers to be damaged during surgery and the patient may describe a sensation of neuropathic pain as these heal. Permanent nerve damage that may be a complication of surgery can lead to chronic pain.

Contracture Following Wound Healing

As a wound heals, the tissue that is reformed may be shortened and less elastic than the tissue that was present before the trauma. This can decrease the range of motion of a joint and there may be obvious deformity at the site. This is frequently seen in areas where there has been tissue damage to a burn. Contractures of muscles and joints can also occur due to immobility. Patients who are immobile for extended periods of time following surgery or trauma are at risk for developing muscle atrophy followed by contracture because of decreased stretching of muscles and use of joints. Contractures can be prevented by having the patient participate in a physical therapy plan that focuses on gentle stretching and mobility exercises while recovery is taking place. If immobility of a specific area of the body will occur during healing, PT can work the patient to gently stretch muscles and joints, if not contraindicated, to prevent contracture formation.

Effects of Multiple Traumatic Injuries on Wound Healing

There are several reactions that occur within the body when multiple trauma injuries occur. The body is triggered to produce more glucose from the glucagon stores within the liver. This is due to the body's increased demands for energy necessary for healing. Electrolyte imbalances are common following tissue destruction and can affect the patient's ability to provide adequate nutrition necessary for wound healing. Oftentimes, there is an increased risk of infection following multiple traumatic injuries because of contaminated wounds. Excessive tissue damage can affect blood flow to an area of trauma which prevents immune factors from entering the region. Excessive blood loss can result in hypovolemic shock and impaired intravascular pressure, which will impair wound healing and could lead to death. Patients who are unconscious following traumatic injury and those who are placed on ventilators are at risk for impaired oxygenation of tissues. Oxygen is necessary for tissue cells to function appropriately and decreased levels of oxygen may decrease the ability of a wound to heal.

Promoting Proper Wound Healing

The CRNFA is involved with surgical wound healing from the time the surgical incision is made through the final healing of the wound. While assisting in surgery, the CRNFA provides adequate tissue retraction and exposure of the surgical site while providing the least amount of tissue trauma possible. This ensures that the surrounding healthy tissues will provide a good environment for adequate wound healing. While closing the surgical incision with skin glue, sutures, or staples, the CRNFA ensures that the wound edges are slightly everted and well-approximated to encourage the development of granulation tissue with wound healing. The CRNFA can educate the patient on proper wound care at home to prevent infection or other complications. Regular wound assessment can also be performed to assess for any changes or the development of a wound infection, dehiscence, or other complication. After wound healing is completed, the CRNFA can re-assess the patient for any long-term complications of surgery and evaluate the patient for any concerns regarding chronic surgical site pain.

Drugs That May Interfere with Proper Wound Healing

Anti-inflammatories will suppress the body's immune response, which can help to decrease pain, but also hinders wound healing. The immune response is necessary to activate specific immune cells to phagocytize bacteria in the area and induce proper wound healing and scar formation. Anti-inflammatories will interfere with this process. This class of medications can also interfere with the formation of protein which is necessary for cell and tissue formation. Anticoagulants will decrease the body's ability to stop bleeding, and may lead to excessive bleeding within the wound. This can develop into a hematoma. Immunosuppressant medications, including steroids can suppress the immune system and impair wound healing. Steroids can also increase the risk of bleeding and elevate glucose levels which will impair proper wound healing. Chemotherapy medications can interfere with the formation of protein and disrupt the replication of cells necessary for tissue growth and wound healing. Radiation treatments can cause changes to skin cells which may prevent cell replication and wound healing.

Clotting and Hemostasis

A blood clot is completely solidified blood which is caused by the action of fibrin and fibrinogen. They are inter-related through a chain of events. Hemorrhage occurs because of some trauma to the outer body or an internal stimulus. This activates the body's clotting system with the migration of platelets and clotting factors to the site. A clot will form and stop the bleeding, if possible, through the action of hemostasis. Coagulation occurs when the blood thickens into a thickened clot using fibrinogen and other proteins. Both hemostasis and coagulation are necessary to control hemorrhage. If functioning properly, this cascade of events can prevent a patient from developing hypovolemic shock and even death from massive hemorrhage. If a clot is present that is not needed, other factors are released to cause fibrinolysis, or the absorption of a clot. This system usually functions appropriately within the body to maintain a normal environment of clotting and fibrinolysis.

Shock Due to Hemorrhage

Shock due to hemorrhage is termed hypovolemic shock. As bleeding occurs, the intravascular volume is decreased. This decreases the amount of circulating blood present and prevents the body's tissues from receiving nutrients that are necessary for proper functioning. This can lead to tissue damage or tissue death. Blood loss in the operating room is estimated by the presence of blood soaked into sponges and on draping materials. The amount of blood in suction canisters can also be measured to determine if the patient is at risk for hypovolemic shock. Once the intravascular volume begins to decrease, the patient's blood pressure will decrease, also. When hypotension becomes severe, death may occur. To treat shock due to hemorrhage, the priority will be to stop the bleeding. This can be done by locating the source of bleeding and repair or clamp off the vessels. IV fluids will be given and, if severe, blood products may be given, also.

Treatment with Blood Products

If the hemoglobin level is decreased, red blood cells (RBCs) may be given. Hemoglobin is attached to RBCs and delivers oxygen to the body's tissues. Administering RBCs increases the hemoglobin level, thus increasing the amount of oxygen circulating in the patient's bloodstream. If a patient has decreased platelets, they are at risk for bleeding during and after surgery. Platelets may be administered to prevent this complication. Further work-up will also probably be needed to determine the cause of the thrombocytopenia. Fresh frozen plasma (FFP) is given to patients who have deficiencies in certain clotting factors. Specific clotting factors can be given, but FFP is useful if these are not available or if the cause of the coagulopathy is unknown. When a patient suffers the loss of a large volume of blood, whole blood will be given to replace all components of the loss blood. The donor blood must be compatible with the patient's blood to prevent a serious reaction.

Controlling Bleeding and Achieving Hemostasis

Direct and Indirect Pressure to Decrease Bleeding

Direct pressure involves using the hands or hemostats to apply pressure directly on the bleeding vessel. This will stop bleeding and allow a clot to form in the area. If there is a lot of bleeding, it may be necessary to hold pressure for several minutes for a clot to form. Another option is to hold a sponge over the area to provide pressure, through this can cause the clot to be torn off the laceration when it is removed. Indirect pressure involves locating the source of the bleeding and attempting to obstruct the flow of blood to the area. Pressure would not be applied directly to the source of the bleeding, but rather to a point just proximal to the hemorrhage to obstruct the blood flow. This is especially helpful when a larger vessel is severed. The vessel is clamped or held at either end, leaving a small amount of tissue at the end. The ends can then be clipped or sutured together for repair.

Hemostatic Staples

When organ resection occurs, such as a hemigastrectomy (partial removal of the stomach), the organ may be sealed closed with staples. This controls bleeding just like using surgical staples for wound closure. Hemostatic staples are available in many different sizes, depending on the surgeon's preference and the type of procedure performed. Studies have been performed to assess the effectiveness of hemostatic staples in securing tissue to prevent hemorrhage during surgery. It has been found that surgical staples provide an adequate means of controlling blood loss during surgery. It is important to fully examine the tissue that has been stapled to ensure there is no residual bleeding. This could lead to hematoma formation among other complications. Other studies have been done to assess the effects of staples when going through an MRI scanner. It has been found that there is no reaction when hemostatic staples are present in a patient receiving a MRI.

Hemostatic Clips

Hemostatic clips are made out of metal or steel wire. They are used seal off the end of a vessel after it has been severed. The clip is smooth on one side and has fine teeth on the other to prevent slipping on tissue. Hemostatic clips can be permanent or can dissolve over time. There are reusable clips that are available for sterilizing after each use to be reused in another patient. A clip is applied far enough away from the end of the vessel to prevent being easily pulled off, but not too far that it leaves excess tissue off the distal end. It is important to ensure the clip is in place before pulling back the special applicator. If the clip is still attached to the applicator, excessive pulling pressure can be placed on it which could cause the clip to be ripped out of place and result in further vessel tissue damage.

Vascular Clamps

Vascular clamps are available in many different shapes and sizes. The clamping ends are usually lined with fine teeth or some type of cushioning material to provide a better grip on the vessel. Ideally, before the clamp is placed on a vessel, the tissue around the area is retracted so that the vessel is completely visualized. The surgeon will usually place the clamp on the vessel, but it is held in place by the CRNFA. The handle of the vascular clamp has a ratcheting closure to prevent accidental slippage. The clamp is usually held by the shaft instead of the ring handles to prevent accidentally loosening the ratcheting. Once the sutures are placed at the end of the vessel, the clamp can be removed. It is important to completely release the clamp off the tissue and then pull the clamp away from the operative site. This prevents any accidental pulling on the vessel which could result in tearing and hemorrhage.

Pneumatic Tourniquets

A pneumatic tourniquet is used to decrease blood flow to an extremity for surgical purposes. A rubber bandage is applied to most distal portion of the extremity and the extremity is elevated to drain as much blood from the limb as possible. The tourniquet is then applied more proximally on the limb to prevent blood from flowing back into the limb. This helps to decrease the flow of blood into the operative site and will help with excessive blood loss during surgery. Extreme care should be taken when applying a pneumatic tourniquet. There is a risk of causing vessel or nerve damage from compression, especially if it is placed at the elbow or knee joints. Padding should be placed under the pneumatic cuff to prevent tissue damage and the cuff should remain smooth at all times to prevent any type of pressure injury to the underlying skin. Any patients who have diseases of the vascular system should not receive a pneumatic tourniquet.

Vascular Tourniquets

An umbilical tape is often used to provide a tourniquet effect on vascular structures. With a blood vessel, the tape is positioned around the vessel and pressure is applied until there is no longer blood flow through the vessel. This is then secured using hemostats. There are also prepackaged vascular tourniquet kits now available that contain all of the equipment necessary to successfully apply a vascular tourniquet. When a purse-string suture is created in a vessel, a tourniquet is frequently used to hold this in place until the sutures are drawn tight. The goal is to provide enough pressure on vessel that blood flow will stop, but not too much pressure so that there is a risk of damaging the tissue that makes up the vessel walls. Whether an umbilical tape or a specialized tourniquet is used to accomplish this goal, the instruments should be removed from the immediate surgical area as much as possible to prevent obstructing the surgeon's view.

Hypothermia

Hypothermia is an extreme decrease in body temperature, down to 95°F or below. When the core body temperature is dropped that low, the circulatory system responds by causing vasoconstriction of all of the vessels in the body. By constricting the blood vessels, bleeding can be decreased. The effects of hypothermia can be quite serious, though, so hypothermia is not recommended to be used to achieve hemostasis. The patient's skin will become very pale as the blood supply to the skin and tissues is decreased with vasoconstriction. In the patient who is awake, there will be signs of confusion with possible loss of consciousness. The respiratory system becomes depressed which leads to shallow breaths and hypoxia. The heart rate will decrease and can lead to cardiac arrest. Cardiac dysrhythmias can occur, also, especially ventricular fibrillation. Isolated areas of the body may be cooled to control bleeding in that area, such as some portions of the GI tract, but caution is used with this to prevent tissue damage.

Hypotension

A decrease in blood pressure will result in a lower risk of bleeding. Surgeries that are known to involve vascular structures or that may cause a large amount of blood loss may require the patient's blood pressure to be decreased during the procedure. The anesthesiologist will administer medications to decrease the patient's blood pressure during surgery, while continually monitoring the vital signs to prevent potential complications. A drop in blood pressure that is severe can lead to organ failure and possibly death. As blood pressure is decreased, there may not be enough blood and nutrients traveling to certain organs, such as the kidneys. This can result in impairment in the organ's function and lead to organ failure. Careful monitoring needs to be maintained to prevent possible irreversible damage that could be life-threatening. Low blood pressure can also be a sign of fluid loss. This can result from excessive bleeding either during surgery or in the postoperative period. IV fluids or blood products may be necessary to prevent hypovolemic shock.

Gelatin Sponges

Gelatin sponges are made from gelatin that has been processed and dried. They can be cut to fit a specific area and may be impregnated with or soaked in a solution containing thrombin. The sponges are placed within the body cavity where the bleeding is occurring and left there to continue to absorb blood. They can hold a good deal of blood and will dissolve after several weeks. Gelatin sponges can hold bacteria if the wound is not sterile. This can result in an infection at the site where the sponge is located. If this were to occur, the patient would need to have the operative site re-opened and the infective material removed. As the sponges absorb more blood, they will expand. Too many sponges or too large of a sponge in an area can cause compression on vessels or organs in the area if they become too large. It is important to cut the sponge to the desired size to be effective but avoid this potential complication.

Thrombin

Thrombin functions by acting on fibrinogen to cause a clot to form in the blood. There are topical thrombin solutions that can be used during surgery to induce clotting. This is used on small vessels. The solution is available ready to use or can be mixed with saline for use. It is usually used by soaking a sponge in the solution and applying the solution to the area where the bleeding is occurring. Applying the solution to large vessels is contraindicated because of the risk of clots forming and traveling through the blood stream. The solution is also never given IV because of its risk of causing multiple blood clots to form within the vascular system which can result in organ failure or death from an embolism. Once the solution has been applied to the area where the bleeding is occurring, excessive pressure or manipulation of the tissue should be avoided to avoid disrupting the clot.

Absorbable Collagen Sponges

Absorbable collagen sponges function very similar to the microfibrillar collagen in that it stimulates the clumping of platelets and the release of substances necessary for the clotting cascade to begin and stop bleeding. It is created from a portion of the connective tissue from a cow. Absorbable collagen sponges were originally designed to be used for bone bleeding, but have found to also be effective at controlling bleeding from small vessels that may be severed during surgery. The absorbable collagen sponges are activated by moisture and should be placed at the site of bleeding suing dry forceps. Rather than taking up to 10 minutes to induce clotting, like the microfibrillary collagen, the absorbable collagen sponges can control bleeding in less than 4 minutes. The collagen sponges remain localized where they are applied. This decreases the risk of future adhesions or vessel and organ compression due to excessive collagen fibers in the area.

Microfibrillar Collagen

Collagen functions to cause platelets to clump together and begin to form a clot. It also stimulates the platelets to release substances that cause the coagulation cascade to begin. Microfibrillar collagen used in surgery is created from the skin tissue of a cow. It is activated by moisture and is placed at the site of bleeding using dry instruments, usually forceps. The collagen is held in place at the site of bleeding using a dry sponge. It may take up to 10 minutes for the collagen to form a clot in the area and the dry sponge should be held in place for that long to ensure adequate clotting. If the bleeding continues after the collagen is applied, the process may be repeated. If excess collagen is left in the area, it can lead to adhesion formation later, especially with intestinal surgery. It can also cause pressure and constriction around blood vessels and other small, tubular structures.

Fibrin Gel

One portion of blood clotting involves thrombin causing fibrinogen to form into fibrin. This results in a clot being formed. Fibrin gel is available and can be applied directly to a site of bleeding to act as a sealant as clots form. It is only effective in small areas of bleeding and will not be effective with copious amounts of bleeding from large vessels. The fibrin gel is activated by mixing it with plasma which can be obtained from the patient or from a blood bank. It is applied along with thrombin to form a strong clot. The two substances are applied from separate syringes because of the quick clotting that will occur when they are mixed together. Because of the quick clotting that occurs, fibrin gel and thrombin should not be applied in a large blood vessel and should never be given IV. This could result in severe clotting and embolism with possible death.

Oxidized Cellulose

Oxidized cellulose is available in gauze or cotton to control bleeding. The materials can be cut to fit a specific area and are applied to small bleeding vessels. It is then held in place with a dry sponge until the bleeding has stopped. The body will absorb the material in about one week. Oxidized cellulose can react with thrombin to prevent thrombin from inducing clotting by working on fibrinogen to activate the clotting cascade. Because of this, it should not be used with thrombin-impregnated products. Oxidized cellulose will also expand as it absorbs blood. Care should be used when using this product because of the risk of applying excess pressure on surrounding vessels, nerves, or organs as the gauze or sponge expands. It should not be used in areas where there is no room for expansion. This material can also hold bacteria and lead to an infection in the operative site. Sterility should be maintained at all times while handling the material.

Epinephrine

Epinephrine has a vasoconstriction effect and can help to decrease bleeding by constricting the blood vessels. Lidocaine and other anesthetics used for providing local anesthesia are available in solution with epinephrine. This is sometimes used as an anesthetizing agent to decrease bleeding before suturing a laceration. Sponges used to absorb blood during surgery can be soaked in epinephrine before being placed in the area of bleeding. This can help by causing vasoconstriction of the vessels in that area. Caution should be used with epinephrine, though. Because it causes constriction of the blood vessels, it can lead to an increase in blood pressure and heart rate and should be avoided in patients with a history of heart disease. Also, it should never be used in the distal portions of any limbs, along with the nose and penis. The vasoconstriction can be quite significant and may lead to tissue death in these smaller areas of tissue.

Albumin

The grafts used in vascular surgeries are made of a material that has many small pores in it. Albumin can be used to cover the grafts and seal those pores. This will prevent blood from leading through the small openings. Clots tend to clump together in areas that have a rougher surface, and the graft prosthesis can feel rough from the multiple pores that present on it. An albumin coating on the graft will make it smoother and prevent platelets from clumping which decreases the risk of clotting of the graft. Albumin solutions are also available to be given intravenously during and immediately after surgery. These help to increase the albumin levels in a patient and increase the colloid pressure in blood. This can help to decrease bleeding and prevent a drastic decrease in hemoglobin, which is monitored for signs of anemia. Studies have been performed that show that patients who receive albumin during surgery have a lower incidence of blood loss.

Bloodless Surgery

Evaluation of the patient before surgery should include reviewing medications for any anticoagulants that may be used, as well as review of lab data to evaluate for the presence of blood dyscrasias that may contribute to blood loss. If surgery is done on an emergent basis, medications should be given to counter the effects of anticoagulants to prevent uncontrollable bleeding. Blood products should also be available in case the patient develops excessive blood during or after surgery. Medications can be administered before surgery that will encourage production of RBCs. These include erythropoietin, certain vitamins, and folic acid. Iron can also be given to increase the RBC and hemoglobin counts. Performing procedures using minimally invasive techniques, if possible, can also help to reduce intra-operative hemorrhage. The skilled use of electrocautery during surgery will also prevent excessive blood loss. Patients who refuse any blood products need to have an obvious identifier on themselves and on their chart stating that they do not wish to receive blood.

Relation of Hypertension to Bleeding

When the blood pressure is elevated, there is a risk of more bleeding during surgery and postoperatively. When blood pressure is high, there is more strain on the vascular system, which can lead to damage to or rupture of the vessel walls. This can result in localized bleeding or a serious complication of a hemorrhagic stroke. Patients who experience pain during a surgical procedure or in the postoperative period can also have a rise in blood pressure. This can contribute to post-op bleeding. Pain should be well-controlled with analgesics to prevent this potentially serious complication. Patients should be screened for uncontrolled hypertension before surgery. All efforts possible should be made to have the patient's blood pressure within the normal range before elective surgery is performed. If a patient requires emergency surgery and the blood pressure is high, treatment with beta blockers and other antihypertensives may be necessary during the perioperative period to prevent serious complications.

Bonewax

Bonewax is created from beeswax and Vaseline. A small piece of it is worked with the hands and pressed into openings in bone tissue to control bleeding from the marrow. It acts solely as a barrier and does not have any biochemical properties. It is minimally absorbed by the body. Bonewax should not be used in areas where bone regrowth is necessary, such as bony sites where a surgical fusion has been performed. Because bonewax is a foreign substance, the body may initiate an inflammatory response against the material and this has been seen in tissues surrounding the location of the bonewax. Because of this, bonewax should be used sparingly to prevent a chronic inflammatory response. If a patient develops a postoperative infection, the presence of bone wax may exacerbate the inflammatory response associated with the infection. Bonewax is not to be reused once it has been opened. Though it is sterile within the package, it cannot be resterilized for future use.

Electrical Circuit, Direct Current, Alternating Currents, Resistance, and Voltage

Electrical circuit is the pathway that electricity follows by following the path of least resistance. It involves the movement of charged particles to move through a conductor and then return to ground. Direct current is the type of electricity that is produced by batteries, static, and lightning. A voltage is created, and possibly stored, until a circuit is completed. Once the circuit is completed, the current flows directly, in one direction. Alternating currents describes electricity that is not provided as a single, constant voltage, but rather as a sine wave that over time starts at zero, increases to a maximum value, then decreases to a minimum value, and repeats. Resistance is the force that opposes the electric current. It is measured in ohms. Voltage is a measurement that depicts the force necessary to cause 1 amplitude to flow through 1 ohm or resistance. Obviously, the higher the voltage means the higher the force of the electricity.

Electrosurgery

Electrosurgery involves applying an electric current to tissue that is bleeding to provide hemostasis. Excessive tissue damage can occur, though, if the electrocautery device is set with an energy level that is too high or nonbleeding tissues are treated with the device. When bleeding is present within the surgical site, pressure should be applied and the exact source of the bleeding should be identified. The electrocautery device should than be applied to the area, using the lowest voltage of electricity necessary to effectively provide hemostasis. A mistake that is frequently made is that electrosurgery techniques are applied over an entire area when there is bleeding instead of just the specific identified vessel that requires cautery. For tissues that tend to bleed quite heavily, such as organ tissue, the electrocautery device may be used for creating the surgical incision. This prevents massive bleeding and the potential resultant effects upon the patient.

Bipolar Electrosurgery

Bipolar electrosurgery is accomplished by using a device that contains both positive and negative poles that are located close together. This allows the electric current to pass from pole to another, rather than through the patient's body. This also prevents a grounding device from being necessary. The instrument is designed like forceps so that the electric current passes through the tissue that is grasped. Bipolar electrosurgery is not very effective against larger bleeding vessels. It is commonly used in surgeries that do not have a large amount of bleeding, such as some neurosurgical procedures. Because the electrical current is contained and not traveling through the patient, it has been recommended with electrical implants, such as a pacemaker or automatic internal cardiac defibrillator. When using a bipolar electrosurgery device, ensure that it is connected correctly to the generator to prevent deliver of a monopolar electric current with resultant tissue damage to the patient.

Electrocautery Pencil

The electrocautery pencil is a relatively small, handheld device that contains a battery which supplies a direct, or simple, current of electricity. This prevents the electric current from leaving the device to travel through the patient. The electrocautery pencil consists of a looped wire at the end of the instrument that is heated by electricity delivered from the battery. This is then used to cauterize bleeding tissue. Because this is based on a simple current of electricity without transmission of the electric current to the patient, a grounding device is not necessary. The drawback to an electrocautery pencil is that it is effective on only small amount of bleeding and cannot be used on larger bleeding tissue. It is frequently used in surgeries that involve small amounts of bleeding, such as eye surgeries. The wire loop on the end of the pencil can easily become adhered to tissue is another drawback to using this device.

Complications of Electrosurgery

Direct Coupling

Direct coupling occurs when the active electrode from the electrosurgery instrument is charged when there is another instrument close by. This is most likely to occur during laparoscopic procedures when the instruments are in a relatively small space. The second instrument will become energized. This energy, or electric current, will then look for a way to travel back to the return electrode. This means that significant patient injury can occur as the electrical current travels through the tissue or body to follow the path of least resistance back to the return electrode. The main injuries seen with this complication are tissue burns. The spark that is generated when this occurs can result in tremendous heat production. If the spark occurs with metal clips it may result in damage or necrosis of the underlying tissue which could cause the clip to fall off the tissue or organ. The electrocautery instrument should never be activated unless all other instruments can be visualized and are not in close proximity.

Insulation Failure

Insulation failure can occur when there are breaks or holes in the insulation. These are usually caused by reprocessing or damage from use. These breaks in the insulation can serve as an alternative pathway for current to leave the electrode as it completes its circuit to the return electrode. If the generator is activated, the current can exit directly into patient tissue that is lying adjacent to the insulation. This can produce significant tissue damage. This can frequently occur outside of the surgical field of vision so the problem may go undetected until there is extensive tissue damage. To prevent an insulation failure from occurring, the insulation should be carefully inspected before every procedure. It should be examined for small cracks and defects, even on brand new units. The generator should not be activated until it is very close to the target tissue. This will ensure that the circuit can be completed through the target tissue without a deviation of the circuit into healthy tissue.

Evolution of Electrosurgery

There is evidence that electrosurgery techniques were being applied to procedures in Egyptian times. The first electrosurgery generator was developed in the 1920s, though, by a biophysicist named William Bovie. This machine used high frequency electrical current that passed through the patient's tissues. Dr. Harvey Cushing, neurosurgery, was the first to use the "Bovie" as it became called to assist in removing a brain tumor. The instrument consisted of two small metal pieces that conducted electricity and were separated by air. This is similar to the function of a spark plug. Dr. Cushing performed over 500 cranial procedures using this device. As more surgeons became familiar with the use of an electrosurgery device, the popularity of the device increased. This new technique allowed the surgeon to perform surgery in less time, with less blood loss, lower infection rates, and decreased tissue damage. Electrocautery is now standard in every operating room around the world.

Preventing Patient Injury During Electrosurgery

When using an electrosurgery instrument, the lowest possible power setting should be used. This prevents accidental burning of tissue. The power setting can be adjusted if it is found the lowest level is not effective. Before beginning a procedure, the instrument should be examined to assess for any breaks or cracks in the insulation. This should not be done only on older, reusable models, but on brand new disposable cauterizers, also. Bipolar electrosurgery is safe because the electrical current is passed through one electrode, through the tissue that is grasped in the instrument, and back into the return electrode. There is no risk of the electrical current traveling through a large portion of tissue without warning. That is if all of the settings on the generator are correct and the patient does not receive a monopolar charge. Be very conscious of there the electrode is placed before using activating the charge. This can prevent contact with other metal instruments within the patient's body, especially with laparoscopic procedures.

Orthopedic

Challenges with Positioning Orthopedic Patient During Surgery

In order for the surgical team to have adequate access to the operative site during orthopedic surgery, careful positioning of the patient is necessary. There is concern that the patient may suffer nerve or vascular damage if positioning is not correct. Most orthopedic surgeries are performed utilizing different types of lateral, prone, and supine positions. Some surgeries are performed with the patient sitting, such as upper cervical surgeries. There is an increased risk of air embolism with this type of positioning and careful monitoring will be done during surgery to ensure the patient is stable. There is also a risk of venous pooling in the lower extremities with this position, which can lead to DVTs and pulmonary embolism. Care should be taken to prevent excessive pressure on bony prominences. Excessive stretching or nerves can also lead to permanent damage, such as a brachial plexus injury with over extension of the upper extremity.

Skin Closure Following Orthopedic Procedures

The material used for wound closure will vary depending upon the location of the surgery. For surgeries performed in areas where there is excessive stress, such as near a large joint, interrupted sutures will usually be used. If there is excessive stretching or bending at the area which causes damage to the sutures, interrupted sutures are more likely to prevent wound dehiscence when compared to continuous sutures. Injury to the area is more likely to damage only a few sutures, rather than the whole line of interrupted sutures, whereas damage to just a few continuous sutures can affect the integrity of the full line of sutures.

Surgical staples may also be used, especially with hip replacement procedures. They provide adequate strength to maintain wound closure and usually do not cause excessive scarring. Absorbable internal sutures may be used to close muscle and soft tissue, but a stronger suture may be necessary if there is an area that receives a good deal of stress. These will remain inside following surgery.

Orthopedic Surgery Instruments

Many orthopedic surgeries require deep access to bone tissue. This may require the use of self-retaining retractors to help prevent excessive fatigue in the hands of the CRNFA and allow his or her hands to be free to assist in surgery. The retractor will need to be removed and repositioned as the surgery progresses. If not placed carefully, the retractor can cause nerve or vessel compression which can lead to permanent tissue damage. Drills and saws are often frequently used to open or sever bone. Proper use of the equipment can decrease the risk of injury, but careful attention to instrument placement before using should be exercised. Special equipment may be worn by the orthopedic surgery team to prevent inhalation of bone dust or small fragments, as well as decrease the risk of bone infection. Special instrumentation can be used that is designed specifically for certain surgeries. This includes joint prostheses, plates, and screws. There are many surgical instrument companies that offer instrumentation to be used in surgery.

Compartment Syndrome

There are two mechanisms involved with the development of compartment syndrome. External pressure on a limb, such as with a restrictive bandage or casting/splinting material, can excessive compression on an anatomical compartment. Internal pressure can result in the increased pressure because of swelling within the tissues. Both causes of compartment syndrome can result in damaging pressure applied to tissue cells, blood vessels, and nerves. This can result in tissue death, pain, and systemic illness. Along with the pain, patients may also describe a numbing sensation. This is due to a combination of decreased blood flow and nerve compression. If this continues, tissue cell death can occur when blood vessels are compressed and permanent nerve damage can occur if the nerve fibers are compressed. Pain or numbness is usually the first symptoms of compartment syndrome that become evident. It is important to remember that the patient may continue to have normal pulses in the affected limb because the arteries are outside of the compartment.

Interventions for Post-Op Patient on Day 1 After Total Knee Replacement

Following a knee replacement, the patient's leg should be in a knee immobilizer when they are resting in bed. This can place the patient at risk for pneumonia and venous stasis leading to a deep venous thrombosis due to inactivity. The patient should perform regular deep breathing and coughing exercises along with incentive spirometry exercises every hour or two. Compression stockings will also be used to encourage blood return from the lower extremities and help to prevent a DVT in the lower leg. Physical therapy will work with the patient on the first day after surgery to assist with transferring from the bed to a chair. Training with a walker will also be started to encourage ambulation. They will also work with the patient to perform exercises in bed to help maintain strength and begin to practice improving mobility of the knee with the new joint prosthesis. At this point, social work will begin working to meet any discharge needs the patient will have.

Cardiac

Exposure of Surgical Site During Cardiac Surgery

As with all surgeries, exposure of the surgical site during cardiac surgery is very important. Fixed retractors are used to hold back the sternum and ribs and provide better access to the chest. These should be carefully placed to prevent unnecessary rib fracture, especially in those patients who may be at risk for osteoporosis. There is also a risk of intercostal nerve damage from retractors. There are specialized retractors available for different types of cardiac procedures, depending upon the anatomic area that requires exposure. During bypass grafting surgery, the CRNFA is responsible for actually holding the heart in his or her hand and carefully retracting it to fully expose the coronary artery to the surgeon. This is done very gently to prevent any damage to the artery or cardiac tissue. The hands should be kept very flat while doing this to provide a clear view of the artery without obstruction.

Interoperative Care for Cardiac Surgery Patients

The patient will be very closely monitored throughout any cardiac procedures. This may require the use of an internal monitoring line, such as an arterial pressure line or CVP line. Transesophageal echocardiography (TEE) may be performed during surgery to more clearly evaluate valve function during surgery. This is especially useful during valve repair or replacement procedures. It can also be used to assess the dimensions of the existing valve when determine which prosthetic valve should be used for replacement. Most cardiac surgeries require the patient be in a supine position. Care should be taken to prevent over stretching of the upper extremities which can lead to a brachial plexus or ulnar nerve injury. All bony prominences should be padded. Excessive pressure should be avoided over the vessels and nerves of the extremities to prevent compromised blood flow or permanent nerve damage. All venous or arterial lines should also be kept free to prevent accidental movement of the lines.

Potential Infection in Cardiac Surgery Patients

The patient and family members or the caregiver should be educated on the signs and symptoms of infection, which can be life-threatening in the cardiac surgery patient. An increase in pain at the surgical site can be an early indicator and this will continue to increase as the infection worsens. If the infection is present throughout the surgical site, the patient may experience some difficulty breathing or an increase in pain with activity. This can occur is the surrounding soft tissue becomes edematous and increases the pressure within the chest cavity. The signs of infection can include an increase in redness surrounding the surgical incision. The area may also feel very warm. Swelling around the incision may increase and there may be noticeable purulent discharge from the wound itself. If the drainage is excessive, there may be a foul odor present. Late signs of infection include fevers >100.5°F and even nausea or vomiting. If an infection becomes systemic, the patient may exhibit signs of mental status changes.

Vein Harvesting During Cardiac Surgery

There are a few different approaches to harvesting veins for bypass grafting. A continuous long incision can be made up the inside of the leg to access the greater saphenous vein, a series of small incisions can be made along the vein's path, or an endoscopic technique can be performed which involves 2 or 3 small incisions to be made. Whichever technique is used, the vein is identified and the proximal end is clamped. The vessel is then carefully dissected away from the surrounding tissues. Small branches off the vein should also be severed. Once it is free, it is removed the leg and carefully placed in a sterile saline bath to be irrigated. It is also carefully flushed to assess for patency. Excessive force should not be used to flush the vein. If any small leaks are identified, fine suture can be used to carefully close these openings. The incisions used to access the vein are then sutured closed using either continuous or interrupted sutures for closure.

General Knowledge/Skills

Supine Position

The supine position is achieved by placing the patient on his or her back and providing comfortable padding underneath all pressure points. The arms should be kept either at the patient's sides or on arm boards that are at a less than 90-degree angle from the operating bed. While in the supine position, the patient's head should be well-padded to prevent pressure being applied to the base of the skull, as well as to prevent the neck from being placed in a misaligned position. Cushioning may also be placed under the legs near the knees to keep the hips and knees slightly flexed. The heels can be subject to pain from persistent pressure during surgery and cushioning should be placed there, also. Consideration should be taken when considering a patient's co-morbidities. Those who suffer from significant respiratory or cardiac illness may have difficulty breathing while in the supine position. This can affect the lung's ability to expand and contract during surgery.

Reverse Trendelenburg Position

The reverse Trendelenburg position is accomplished by placing the patient in a supine position and tilting the table so that the lower extremities are down and the head is up. The patient should be safely and securely strapped to the table to prevent falls. This surgery is useful in decreasing blood flow to the head and upper body. It can also help to prevent the abdominal organs from placing pressure under the diaphragm, thereby increasing the lung's ability to maximally expand with respiration. Because the blood return to the heart is decreased in the position, DVT precautions should be followed to prevent formation of blood clots in the lower extremities. Pneumatic compression stockings may be used to provide compression of the veins in the lower extremities to prevent stasis of blood. This position may be useful in a situation in which blood flow to the upper body is desired or to help move the abdominal organs down when performing surgery in the upper abdomen or around the diaphragm.

Trendelenburg Position

The Trendelenburg position is similar to the supine position, but the table is tilted so the head is lower than the rest of the body. This can help to move the abdominal organs cephalad, or toward the head, to help with abdominal or pelvic surgery. This position also helps to raise a patient's blood pressure and increase blood return to the heart. If a patient requires a central line, the Trendelenburg position can help distend the veins in the neck, making this an easier task. For surgery that will be performed in the lower half of the body, the Trendelenburg position can help decrease blood loss by slowing down blood loss from the surgical site. Patients who suffer from chronic lung disease may not be able to tolerate the Trendelenburg position. The movement of the abdominal organs against the diaphragm can decrease the lung's ability to expand with respirations. The increased blood flow to the brain may also be contraindicated in those patients who suffer from head trauma.

Prone Position

The prone position is when the patient is face-down on the table. Extreme care needs to be taken to ensure that the patient is safely rotated to the prone position after he or she is intubated in the supine position. Several people are involved to assist with rotating the patient. Once the patient has been rolled into a prone position, the first priority is to ensure the airway did not become dislodged. The position would need to be moved out of the prone position if re-intubation is necessary. Cushioning rolls will also be placed along either side of the patient to cushion the shoulders, sides, and hips. A pillow may be placed under the abdomen and pelvis. The arms are extended onto arm boards and cushioned to prevent excessive pressure on bony prominences. A molded cushion is placed under the face to prevent pressure on the nose and chin. The eyes must also be protected to prevent cornea damage.

Lithotomy Position

The lithotomy position is achieved by laying the patient supine and flexing the hips and knees with the legs elevated. The legs are supported with stirrups that may support portions of the legs or the whole legs. Ankle straps may also be used to help elevate the lower extremities. The biggest concern with this position is the risk of nerve damage in the lower extremities. The sciatic nerve, the largest nerve in the body, can be overly stretched and this can lead to change in motor function as well as sensory deficits in the lower extremities. The sciatic nerve divides to become the common peroneal and tibial nerves. The common peroneal nerve is responsible for dorsiflexion of the feet and damage to this nerve may result in foot drop. Other nerves can be damaged that will affect various parts of the lower extremities with both motor and sensory function. The lithotomy position is frequently used for gynecologic and urologic surgery, and any other procedures that require exposure to the perineum.

Sitting Position

The sitting position is rarely used now because of multiple complications that can occur. The patient is intubated while supine and then slowly manipulated into a sitting position by the OR staff. The arms and hands are rested in the lap in a relaxed position and the legs are slightly elevated with the knees slightly flexed. The patient is secured to the table to prevent movement during surgery and the head is affixed in place with screws into the skull that holds the head in a brace. This position has been used for skull base surgeries of the posterior fossa. There is an increased risk of an air embolism because of the variant in pressure between the intravascular space and the external environment. When the venous sinus is opened, the possibility exists that air can enter and cause a potentially fatal air embolism. There is also a risk for DVTs in the lower extremities and compression stockings may be used to prevent venous stasis and potential clotting.

Lateral Decubitus Position

Left or right lateral decubitus positioning is when the patient is positioned on their left or right side, respectively. The patient is intubated while supine and then rolled onto the necessary side. A cushion is placed on the table that runs the length of the patient's body. Cushions are also placed under the side that is against the table to accommodate chest expansion with respirations, and between the legs to maintain hip alignment. Cushions must also be placed under the head and neck to maintain cervical alignment. The lateral decubitus position is frequently used with procedures that require entry through the side of the patient. This can be used with thoracic surgeries, such as lung lobectomies, or during kidney removal or transplantation. This position does not affect the patient's ability to expand the lungs during respiration and the abdominal organs are not applying pressure under the diaphragm which can impede respirations.

Patient Education of Preoperative Process

The whole surgical experience can be a little overwhelming and can induce some anxiety in the patient. The CRNFA can ease this anxiety by educating the patient on what to expect during the preoperative period. The patient should be educated on the necessary lab work and other testing that will be completed prior to surgery. This can usually be completed a few days before surgery. The patient will usually need to be at the hospital very early the morning of surgery, if not admitted in the days beforehand. Clear instructions should be given explaining where the patient will need to go when they arrive at the hospital, what will be done the morning of surgery (IV started, anesthesia evaluation, etc.), and how long the surgery should last. The patient's family should also be educated on how long they can expect to be waiting for surgery to be completed. Any process that is in place regarding informing the family about the progress of surgery should also be explained to them

Patient Education of Post-Op Pain Management

A patient's pain level has said to be the "fifth vital sign." More and more attention has been focused on the frequent assessment and treatment of a patient's pain in order to keep them as comfortable as possible following surgery. The CRNFA should be realistic and honest when explaining to the patient the amount of pain they should expect following surgery. This will help the patient so that they are not surprised with how much pain they have following surgery. The patient should be encouraged to utilize pain medications that are provided to them following surgery. They should not feel that they need to "tough it out" to avoid pain medications. The patient should also be educated about the myth that using pain medication for a short time following surgery will cause them to become an addict.

The CRNFA can also educate the patient on the proper time to use pain medication prophylactically, such as before increased activity with physical therapy, to avoid an increase in pain.

Postoperative Infection

An infection can start with some mild redness (erythema) and swelling (edema) around the incision site. There may also be some warmth. The patient may complain of pain or tenderness with palpation around the incision. They may also have a fever or complain of generalized symptoms of nausea, vomiting, fatigue, or general malaise. After the initial signs of an infection appear, a discharge may develop from the incision with purulent drainage. This can range in color from yellow to green or greenish-blue. This may also have an odor to it. The skin around the incision may be indurated with a firm feeling when palpated. Infection is diagnosed by the clinical appearance, but cultures can also be done to define which bacterium is responsible for the infection. When a culture is done, a sensitivity test will also be completed to assess which antibiotic will be the most affective at treating the infection.

Wound Healing

Pathophysiology

When the body tissues sustain some type of injury, the body's clotting cascade is immediately activated. This helps to promote clot formation at the site of injury and minimize blood loss. The immune system then responds by sending specific cells to destroy any foreign material that may be present. This process can last up to three days. After this phase is completed, specialized cells called fibroblasts travel to the area to lay down fibrin to help with healing. Epithelial cells and collagen are also present to help with tissue regeneration and healing. This phase will continue for several weeks while the area of injury heals and a scar is formed. Over the next several months to years the scar will continue to reshape itself and go through a phase called remodeling. This causes the scar to contract and contractures of the tissue can occur if proper care is not taken to provide splinting and range of motion to the area.

Skin Grafts to Promote Healing

Skin grafts are used to form the superficial layer of the wound when there is extensive tissue damage that prevents wound healing. The skin is either from a donor or can be harvested from the patient. The graft is a very thin layer of skin that does not contain its own blood supply. The graft can be split thickness which involves the outer layer of skin and part of the dermis, or second layer, or it can be a full thickness graft which includes all of the first two layers of skin. The graft is placed over the open wound and the blood supply from the recipient will function to heal the wound by incorporating the graft into the layers of tissue. The first few days of healing following placement of the skin graft are crucial to ensure the graft is not moved and that the blood supply is not compromised. Collections of blood can form under the graft so a small drain may be placed to prevent this complication.

Patient Education on Wound Care

The patient should know their limitations when a wound is going through the healing process. This should include information on keeping the wound clean and how it should be properly cleansed. Inform the patient of any activity limitations, such as excessive movement or bending of the portion of the body where the wound is located. Also provide guidelines for the patient for elevation or ice application to help decrease edema. Explain to the patient or caregiver how the dressing over the wound should be applied and how frequently it should be changed. Provide the patient with the adequate materials to change the dressing or advise them where these supplies can be purchased. The patient should be educated on the signs and symptoms of infection. Also advise the patient to monitor their temperature to assess for any fever which may indicate an infectious process. Provide the patient with a phone number to call if there is concern that there is a problem with the wound.

Cellulitis

Cellulitis is an infection that occurs in a wound and involving the surrounding soft tissues. It is characterized by edema, erythema, warmth, and discomfort surrounding the wound. The patient may or not develop a fever with cellulitis. A white blood cell count may be elevated, as well as an elevation in the erythrocyte sedimentation rate, though this test is specific for cellulitis. Cellulitis is usually called by a form of strep bacteria, though other organisms can also be responsible for the infection. Treatment will include oral antibiotics, though IV antibiotics may be administered if the infection is extensive. Incision and drainage of the infection is rarely used. If significantly extensive, incision and debridement may be necessary if there is concern that devitalized tissue is present. Cellulitis infections can become systemic and lead to sepsis if they are not treated and if the patient's immune system is not able to ward off the spreading bacteria. This can be determined by testing blood cultures for any growth of bacteria.

Tetanus

Though uncommon, tetanus can develop following the infection of a traumatic wound with *C. tetani* bacteria. This can be life-threatening if left untreated. Most patients will develop anxiety and irritability along with spastic and rigid muscles. This first becomes evident in the musculature surrounding the wound. It can progress to include more muscle groups and may even affect the diaphragm which can lead to respiratory arrest. This muscle spasm is what has given the disease the nickname "lockjaw." Tetanus vaccination is available and is given by IM injection. Patients can receive a booster of this every 10 years. If a patient suffers some type of trauma and has a wound, ask about their vaccination status. If they are unsure when the last tetanus shot was given, it is advisable to administer a booster at that time. Patients who developed tetanus are treated with tetanus immunoglobulin. They may be intubated with ventilatory support if necessary.

Lymphangitis

Lymphangitis is a bacterial infection that affects the lymph system. Red streaking will be seen under the skin extending off of lymph vessels and enlarged lymph nodes, or lymphadenopathy, will be present. Blistering may also develop in the skin overlying the infection. The patient will usually have a fever with lymphangitis and may develop an elevated white blood cell count as the infection progresses. An abscess may develop in the area of infection or signs and symptoms of cellulitis may be present. Lymphangitis can develop into a serious systemic infection if not treated promptly and appropriately with antibiotics. The source of the infection should be identified and treated, also. Streptococcus is the most common bacteria to cause lymphangitis. It is possible to biopsy a small portion of affected, inflamed tissue to definitively diagnose the bacteria responsible for the infection so that appropriate treatment can be started. However, treatment should not be delayed because of the risk of rapid development of systemic infection.

Meleney's Ulcer

Meleney's ulcer is a type of progressive gangrene that can involve large areas of tissue with necrotizing ulcers. These ulcers are caused by both Staph and Strep bacteria. The ulcers appear brown at their core with purple and red tissue surrounding the ulcers. They will have a foul-smelling discharge. Like gas gangrene, this type of ulcerating infection can become systemic with possible life-threatening consequences. Patients with Meleney's ulcer must undergo extensive debridement and removal of infected tissue. This can leave a wide, gaping wound depending on the involvement of infection. This will be left open to heal by secondary intention with the formation of granulation tissue within the wound bed. Scarring may be extensive after wound healing has completed. Hyperbaric oxygen treatments have been shown to be very effective in promoting healthy, rapid wound healing. Antibiotics may be necessary for treatment if it has been determined that there is systemic involvement.

Gas Gangrene

Gas gangrene is a potentially life-threatening infection that can occur in a wound. It is caused by the Clostridium bacteria. The patient will have dead tissue and muscle present in the wound with a foul-smelling discharge. There may be gas bubbles present in the discharge and they may be palpated around the wound. Patients with gas gangrene can develop septic shock quite rapidly with a decrease in blood pressure, increased heart rate, difficulty breathing, and mental status changes. They may have only a low-grade fever. Treatment of gas gangrene involves emergency surgical debridement. All of the devitalized tissue and muscle must be removed in the area. This can result in an extensive operative wound, but it is imperative that there are clean wound edges to allow for proper tissue healing. This type of wound will often be left open to heal by secondary intention. This is necessary to prevent closure of the wound with possible residual bacteria in the wound bed that can result in reformation of an infection.

Actinomycosis

The bacteria *Actinomyces* is usually found in the nose and throat and does not normally cause infections in healthy individuals. When a person undergoes some type of trauma or surgery, such as oral surgery, the bacteria can form an abscess that appears as a hard red-purple mass. This frequently occurs along the jaw line, but occur at other sites as well. The abscess will eventually rupture at the skin surface and residual sinus tracts will be present draining a purulent exudate that contains granules of sulfur. If severe, the wound may need to be surgically debrided and left open to heal. Antibiotics are necessary to eradicate the bacteria and therapy may last up to one year depending on the extensive nature of the infection. If left untreated, the bacterial infection can spread to the meninges and lead to meningitis or spread systemically and lead to sepsis, which can lead to death.

Creutzfeldt-Jakob Disease

Creutzfeldt-Jakob disease affects the nervous system and is progressive, leading to death. Its presenting symptoms are similar to those seen with mad cow disease, but the exact cause of the disease is unknown. It is viral in nature and the only known cause is by direct contact with infected tissue. It is thought that after exposure, the virus will sit dormant for a long time, up to 40 years, before symptoms develop. There is a higher prevalence of the disease in certain ethnic groups, such as certain groups of those of Jewish descent, but know known controlled risk factors. There have been documented cases in which transmission occurs through contaminated medical equipment. The virus that causes Creutzfeldt-Jakob disease is very resilient to standard cleansing procedures and can remain on medical equipment used in invasive procedures. It is higher in concentration within the tissues that make up the nervous system, so equipment used during invasive procedures involving this tissue should be sterilized utilizing specific guidelines known to eradicate the virus.

Measures Taken with Instruments and Equipment to Prevent Transmission

Any procedures that will be performed on those patients suspected to have Creutzfeldt-Jakob disease must be sterilized using specific guidelines to kill the virus. Disposable items should be used during the procedure when possible, but even these should be sterilized before disposal. Any skin exposure to the infected tissues should be followed by immediate cleansing of the area with bleach. If there is exposure to blood or body fluids not found in the tissues in which infection has occurred, the area should be thoroughly washed with soap and water. Instruments that are reusable should be soaked in sodium hydroxide for at least one hour. These should then be autoclaved before they are handled. The operating room should be cleansed using a bleach solution to kill any viral cells that may linger on surfaces. All linens and any other objects that came in contact with the patient should be placed in proper disposable bags so that they are recognized as biohazard materials.

Orthopedic Patient Education

Education for each patient will vary depending on the specific procedure performed. All patients should be told honestly before surgery how much pain to expect during the rehabilitation process. They should also have some expectations set regarding how long the convalescence period will last and if any special therapies will be necessary after surgery. Following surgery, patients should be encouraged to deep breath and cough to prevent respiratory complications. Instructions should be given regarding the amount of movement that should be performed and any specific movements that should be avoided. The patient should also be given some sort of time frame in which their mobility can be increased, if possible. Any wound care instructions should be carefully relayed to the patient or caregiver along with the potential signs and symptoms that occur with infection. The patient should also be instructed in using any devices, such as crutches, a walker, or cane. The patient should understand how to safely use their pain medication without over medicating or under medicating themselves.

Cardiac Surgery Patient Education

The patient should fully understand the procedure he or she will be undergoing, along with postoperative expectations regarding pain and that rehabilitation that will be necessary. Education should also include the long-term prognosis for this patient, along with any lifestyle changes that will need to take place. The patient will most likely need to change their eating habits, exercise routine, and some activities in order to obtain the most benefit from the surgery and to increase their odds of survival. In the immediate postoperative period, the patient should be shown how to perform regular deep breathing and coughing exercises, along with incentives spirometry exercises, every hour. It is important to show the patient how to brace or cushion their chest while doing this to help decrease pain. The family or caregiver should also be included in this education process. The patient should be closely monitored for signs of depression or anxiety as they go through this major life changing event.

Stress-Coping Model

Stressful stimuli can be internal or external. Internal stressors would be the direct result of a physical medical condition or mechanical changes due to surgery. External stressors are from psychosocial factors, such as family or financial concerns. When exposed to these stimuli, the body undergoes both psychological and chemical changes. This can cause a physical response in the body, such as the presence of symptoms that are seen with specific conditions, such as chest pain with an acute myocardial infarction, or nervousness and tearfulness with anxiety. As the body is continually confronted with these stimuli, these changes continue to occur. The CRNFA can continually evaluate these stimuli and the reaction that the patient will have to them. This can help to aid the patient in developing constructive coping behaviors to prevent these symptoms from developing, as well as to formulate appropriate medical treatments to properly treat any symptoms that develop.

Erikson's Development Stages for Adults

The Early Adult stage occurs from the early 20s to the mid-40s. During this time frame, a person is dealing with intimacy versus isolation issues. This is the time when people are looking for a mate, having children, and forming a solid career. Life goals are also established during this stage. The Middle Adult stage occurs from the mid-40s to the mid-60s. A person is struggling with issues of generativity versus stagnation during this phase. During middle age, most people are coping with the physical changes of aging, along with dealing with career issues and retirement. Parents in this stage often have children leaving home to start their own families and the "empty nest syndrome" can occur. The Late Adult stage occurs after the age of 60 until death. A person is struggling with issues of integrity versus despair. Physical changes occur and many people are faced with the death of friends and family members. Most people retire during this stage and develop new hobbies and other intellectual stimulating activities.

Professional Practice

Development of RN First Assistant Position

During the Crimean War in the mid-1850s, Florence Nightingale enforced strict guidelines to help prevent surgical infection and promote cleanliness in the operating room. She also helped to educate her staff on care of the surgical incision to help prevent complications. During the Civil War, the work of Dorothea Dix and Clara Barton helped to break down the barriers to women working in healthcare. These nurses were able to show surgeons how valuable the nurse is in the operative room and following surgery when providing post-operative care. World War I and World War II both saw nurses taking a more independent role by performing wound care, including wound debridement, on their own. The Vietnam War saw much more seriously wounded soldiers, as well as many more wounded soldiers, which opened the door for more opportunities for nurses in a surgical role. Surgeons were more appreciative of the value of surgical nurses and the assistance they can provide in a busy operating room.

RN First Assistant Role Since World War II

Education has expanded the role of the RN First Assistant since the mid-1940s. Accredited nursing programs now offer more time in their curriculum focusing on the role of the Registered Nurse in the operating room. This has served to further educate Registered Nurses on surgical procedures, the role of the First Assistant, and the care of the surgical patient. With a broader education base, RN First Assistants are better prepared to appropriately assess the patient before surgery, assist during surgery, and evaluate the patient for complications immediately after surgery. Registered Nurses have also gained more respect from surgeons. More surgeons have realized the important role that RN First Assistants can serve in the operating room and have come to respect their role and appreciate their participation as a member of the operating team. Finally, RN First Assistants have gained the privilege of a distinct certification that is necessary to hold the title. The certification exam must be passed by a Registered Nurse in order to carry the title of CRNFA.

Evolution of Education to Fulfill Need for RN First Assistants

In the past, nurses were trained in providing direct patient care during illness or after surgery. With the development of more advanced surgical treatment options for patients, it became evident that more training needed to be provided to nurses in order for them to be a more effective member of the operating room team. Nursing education programs incorporated some time for training in operating room nursing, as well as providing clinical time for the student nurse to become more familiar with the operating room. As surgeries become more specialized, it became evident that operating room nursing staff would also need to accommodate this trend toward specialization. With the changes seen in medicine today, CRNFAs are even in more demand. Certification is offered for nurses to specialize as CRNFAs and earn the title of a Certified Registered Nurse First Assistant. This indicates the nurse has undergone the specialized training necessary, as well as passed a board exam, in order to earn that certification.

Future Opportunities for RN First Assistants

As the value of RN First Assistants has become appreciated, the financial benefits of utilizing CRNFA services have also become known. Physicians and hospitals began receiving payment from insurance companies after certification was initiated in 1992. Not all states recognize this, but more and more states are enacting guidelines for insurance reimbursement. The focus for the future will be on advancements of the RN First Assistant receiving insurance payment for services nationwide. This will come with the increased awareness of improved patient care and an increase in productivity. More research is being done to look at the areas of surgical care that are better improved by utilizing RN First Assistants. This not only affects financial areas, such as an increase in cost effectiveness, but helps to improve overall patient satisfaction with their surgical experience. More institutions and physicians are using CRNFAs to help provide better care for their patients. As more and more RN First Assistants are used, goals of the profession will become more attainable.

Sunset Law and Sunset Audit

The sunset law is present in most states. It is responsible for monitoring the boards of a state to verify that they are legitimate. There are some boards that are formulated that do not have formalized meetings or do not have enough member or participants to actually form a board. A sunset audit involves a thorough investigation into all aspects of a particular board. This includes its actions, activities, financial situation, and any changes that have been made in the past. A sunset audit can be helpful to its members because it helps to ensure that a board is functioning in the way they should be with its member's best interests in mind. If it is found that a board is not operating for whatever reason, then a motion may be made to dissolve the board. This is done at the legislative level of state government and final approval is received by the state governor.

State Nursing Board

Each state has a nursing practice act that outlines the rule and regulations that must be followed by each nurse practicing within that state. The role of the state nursing board is to enforce those rules to protect patients from negligent practice. The state nursing board is also responsible for the license of individual nurses. This involves issuing the certification exam for nurses and verifying that all nurses have completed the appropriate training necessary to work in that state as a nurse. State nursing boards regulate nursing education programs and verify that these programs meet the standard requirements to be considered an accredited school of nursing. They are also responsible for auditing these programs to ensure that all responsibilities of that program to the nursing student are being met.

In a situation in which a nurse has failed to comply with or has violated the rules of the state's nurse practice act, the state board of nursing is responsible for disciplining, and possibly revoking the license, of the nurse.

Hospital Credentialing of Nonphysician Providers

Obtaining individual hospital privileges to practice by a nonphysician provider (Physician Assistant, Nurse Practitioner, or RN First Assistant) symbolizes the important of this role as a member of the healthcare team. Hospital privileges provide the clinician with autonomy and an increased level of respect by being recognized by the governing body of an institution. This also helps to open the door for nonphysician providers in expanding their role. If functioning on a contractual basis, the nonphysician provider can broaden their area of practice to provide patient care to more people. There has been resistance to nonphysician providers receiving hospital privileges in different areas of the country, but this is changing in most areas. As more providers are aware of the benefits of offering this service to their patients, more institutions are recognizing the importance of offering practice privileges to these clinicians. With healthcare changes, the use of nonphysician providers has also proven to be much more cost effective.

Credentialing Requirements for Facilities

Every institution will vary somewhat in their requirements for practice privileges within their facility, but there are some basic requirements that almost all will require. The clinician must have graduated from an accredited educational program of study for their profession. This is a requirement for the person to complete the national certification exam and state licensing procedures. Proof of current certification and licensing must also be provided. Evaluation by peers is almost always necessary, also. This may be a generic form to be completed or may include specific questions to be answered. The references utilized for this information should be people with whom the clinician has worked closely with and those who can attest to their excellence in practice. All healthcare professions require some type of continuing education to be completed on an annual or bi-annual basis. Proof of this education may be required for verification that educational requirements have been met.

RN First Assistants Contribution to Facility's Performance Goals

Multiple studies have been done, and are still being done, to study the effectiveness of the RN First Assistant as a vital member of the operating room team. It has been shown that patient satisfaction is much higher with the use of CRNFAs which can be in part because of increased productivity. Increased productivity can increase the number of surgical cases performed in a given time period, which has obvious financial benefits for the institution. With the CRNFA performing more clinical duties, the physician's time is not as constrained which can give physicians more time that is necessary to perform other duties they need to complete. This can help in decreasing turnover time in the operating room as well as increasing the productivity of the surgeon. The thoroughness of an RN First Assistant can also help to increase communication among the surgical team which aids in providing better quality care for the patient.

Change in Doctor-Nurse Relationship

In the past, nurses functioned to provide patient care by carrying out orders written by doctors. They were expected to not question these orders and to strictly perform patient care without initiating any interventions on their own without an order. This began to change as nurses, especially in the operating room, gained more respect during World War I. It began to become clear that nurses could be trained to provide adjunct care during surgery. With World War II, operating room nurses began to function more independently and physicians began to see the importance of having an effective nurse as an assistant during surgery. About 10 years after the war ended, the Association of Operating Room Nurses was formed to provide autonomy for these nurses. This was followed by the development of the Registered Nurse First Assistant. Now the CRNFA is an invaluable member of the operating room team. Surgeons depend on the CRNFA to provide patient care and facilitate an efficient surgical procedure.

Collaborative Practice

A collaborative practice is one in which all of the professionals who are treating a patient for specific problems work together to achieve a common goal. In healthcare, this goal would be to improve the patient's overall health and functionality. With the changes in healthcare, and more specialization, the collaborative practice has expanded to include many people. The CRNFA is one person treating the patient, but must work closely with all others for the betterment of the patient. The CRNFA can help facilitate this by openly communicating with the other team members. For example, if a patient is undergoing orthopedic surgery and it is known they will require physical therapy services while in the hospital, the CRNFA can discuss this in advance with the PT personnel to establish goals for the patient and develop a plan of care. If the patient will require placement in a skilled nursing facility to receive more care and rehabilitation following surgery, the CRNFA can discuss this with Social Work in advance.

Primary Nursing

Primary nursing is the direct nursing care that is provided to patients without the assistance of any other specialties. Nurses have been given more independence to formulate a treatment plan to meet the individual patient's needs, which has helped to increase control of their practice. Primary nursing has also helped to provide better patient care by encouraging nurses to practice more independently while providing patient care, yet maintaining increased accountability for their actions. With nursing care focusing more on the patient and their needs, the physicians can focus on medical care of the patient. Nurses can formulate a treatment plan that will work with the physician's plan of care to ensure total treatment of the patient. With this increase in nursing responsibility, physicians have moved toward an attitude of increased respect for nursing care and have come to value the care that nurses provide for the patients. This has also helped to increase patient satisfaction with the healthcare experience.

National Joint Practice Committee

The National Joint Practice Committee was established in the early 1970s. Its goal was to bring together nurses and physicians in order to provide better patient care through communication between the two groups. It encouraged collaboration between both nurses and doctors to establish a synergistic relationship that would benefit the patient.

This also served for nurses and physicians to establish guidelines and specific practice competency that should be met in order to meet the patient's needs. Physicians began to rely on the nurses to provide sound clinical judgment when possible, and the nurses were able to provide a more thorough assessment and evaluation of the patient to assist the physician. This also helped nurses to gain more independence and accountability for their practice. The National Joint Practice Committee had very positive results that are still seen today in patient care. It dismantled in the early 1980s once its goals were met.

The team of professionals who work in the operating room must function well together in order for surgery to be completed as efficiently as possible. It is advisable the staff in the OR establish a joint practice committee so that each healthcare profession can have representation to discuss concerns or ideas for improvement in the OR. For example, a nurse representative on the joint practice committee can bring forth some concerns that other OR nurses may have regarding documentation or patient care. The surgeon member of the committee may have some ideas for improvement from a surgeon's point of view. The idea is to have multi-specialty input to improve the overall operative experience for the patient to ensure the surgical procedure is managed as efficiently and effectively as possible. Areas of concern should also be addressed, as well as new protocols or operating systems discussed to improve work effectiveness. This provides a means by which each specialty can communicate their concerns or ideas to the OR staff.

CRNFA Skills to Function Successfully

The CRNFA must first have the technical knowledge necessary to help with surgical assisting. This includes experience with performing specific procedures and manual skills, as well as familiarity with the pertinent anatomy and physiology. Because the CRNFA functions as an extra set of hands for the surgeon, they must be able to work fluidly with the surgeon. With time, the surgeon's preferences will be known which will help to anticipate the next step to be performed during a surgery. The CRNFA must be level-headed in emergency situations and flexible enough to "go with the flow" when changes arise. Medicine is not an exact science and the plan of care may change unexpectedly. These changes should be expected and dealt with appropriately. Most importantly, the CRNFA should recognize their limitations and weak areas in order to protect themselves and their patients. It is always safer to admit you do not know something than try to guess and place the patient in harm's way.

Challenges Faced in Orthopedic Surgery

The field of orthopedic surgery, as with most specialized medicine, is constantly changing. New surgical techniques are regularly being introduced and the CRNFA must stay up to date and educated on these techniques. This includes undergoing regular training sessions with surgical equipment representatives, learning from attending surgeons, and performing individual reviews of printed studies that have been performed. The CRNFA must also consider the patient's multiple co-morbidities that may be present before undergoing a large surgery, such as a joint replacement. For example, a patient with vascular disease should be assessed for risks of DVT formation following surgery because of their vascular compromise combined with possible decreased activity levels following surgery. Patient education may also be the responsibility of the CRNFA to prepare the patient for what to expect following surgery. This includes instructions on wound dressing changes and limitations in mobility. Good communication is key in aiding the patient's recovery. This includes discussions with PT, OT, and social work for patient placement.

CRNFA Practice Test

Want to take this practice test in an online interactive format?
Check out the online resources page, which includes interactive practice questions and much more:
mometrix.com/resources719/crnfa

1. The patient would most likely be placed in the lithotomy position for which type of surgery?

a. Spinal
b. Cranial
c. Gynecological
d. Thoracic

2. Retractors are used to:

a. cut or separate tissue.
b. remove tissue or other materials.
c. close the severed ends of a vessel.
d. hold back wound edges.

3. The meninges of the spinal cord consist of:

a. the dura mater, the spina mater, and the pia mater.
b. the dura mater, the arachnoid mater, and the pia mater.
c. the dura mater and the pia mater.
d. the dura mater, the arachnoid mater, and the spina mater.

4. The left lung is divided into:

a. superior and inferior lobes.
b. upper, lower, and medial lobes.
c. superior, middle, and inferior lobes.
d. costal and medial lobes.

5. Which of the following is an example of a Grade I neurological surgical complication?

a. Draining wound infection
b. Cerebral hemorrhage
c. Transient confusion that does not require therapy
d. TIA requiring anti-coagulant therapy

6. You are instructing a student nurse on the Brush-Stroke method. What do you teach her?

a. Scrub nails of one hand 10 strokes; each side of each finger, starting with the thumb, 10 strokes; the back of the hand 10 strokes; the palm of the hand 10 strokes; the arm 20 strokes for each 1/3 and each side, to 2 inches above the elbow.
b. Scrub nails of one hand 20 strokes; each side of each finger, starting with the thumb, 30 strokes; the back of the hand 30 strokes; the palm of the hand 30 strokes; the arm 30 strokes for each 1/4 and each side, to 4 inches above the elbow.
c. Scrub nails of one hand 30 strokes; each side of each finger, starting with the thumb, 20 strokes; the back of the hand 20 strokes; the palm of the hand 20 strokes; the arm 20 strokes for each 1/3 and each side, to 2 inches above the elbow.
d. Scrub the thumb 30 strokes; the back of the hand 20 strokes; the palm of the hand 20 strokes; the arm 20 strokes for each 1/4 and each side, to 2 inches above the elbow.

7. Surgical patients who are considered obese are more susceptible to the following EXCEPT:

a. shearing.
b. infection.
c. allergy to anesthesia.
d. tissue hypoxia.

8. A common side effect of midazolam (Versed) is:

a. hypotension.
b. urinary tract infection.
c. dehydration.
d. diarrhea.

9. During what phase of wound healing does granulation occur?

a. Proliferative phase
b. Remodeling phase
c. Inflammatory phase
d. Cytokine phase

10. Which type of suture is absorbable?

a. Surgical silk
b. Surgical cotton
c. Collagen
d. Nylon

11. Which of the following is an example of a clean-contaminated wound?

a. Gunshot wound to the abdomen
b. Viscera perforation
c. Breast biopsy
d. Hysterectomy

12. An infant has approximately which percentage of body water content?

a. 60%
b. 95%
c. 45%
d. 70%

13. Ms. Jones dons her gloves by handling the gloves through the sleeve of her gown and inserting her hands into the gloves as she pushes her arm through the cuff opening. Which gloving technique is she using?

a. Assisted-gloving technique
b. Closed-gloving technique
c. Open-gloving technique
d. Cuffed-gloving technique

14. All of the following are common signs and/or symptoms associated with malignant hyperthermia EXCEPT:

a. hypoxia.
b. tachycardia.
c. vomiting.
d. cardiac dysrhythmias.

15. Which of the following is an example of a preventative measure taken in order to reduce pressure ulcers in the operative patient?

a. Place a pillow under the lower legs in order to raise the heels off the OR bed.
b. Ensure the patient remains immobile during the procedure.
c. Lift the patient every few minutes.
d. Place the patient's legs in stirrups.

16. What is the first action that should be taken immediately after an accidental needle stick?

a. Wash the exposed area with water and soap or disinfectant.
b. Go to the emergency department.
c. Put ointment on the wound.
d. Call for help.

17. Which of the following can help prevent lens fogging during an endoscopic procedure?

a. Blowing on the lens
b. Wiping the lens with a sterile defogging solution
c. Warming the lens under the patient prior to insertion
d. Soaking the endoscope in warm tap water

18. Wound debridement:

a. closes a wound.
b. removes dead tissue from a wound.
c. cleans a wound.
d. keeps a wound moist.

19. A risk associated with prolonged prone positioning includes:

a. substantial blood loss.
b. wound dehiscence.
c. eye injury including temporary or permanent blindness.
d. increased post-operative pain.

20. Which stitches are tied in a continuous suture?

a. Every third stitch
b. The first and last stitch
c. Every other stitch
d. The last stitch

21. The nurse explained to the patient that after her needle biopsy of the liver she should maintain bed rest. The patient questioned why she must maintain bed rest following the procedure. What should the nurse teach the patient?

a. Since anesthesia will be given, bed rest will prevent the patient from falling down.
b. There is a high risk of bleeding post biopsy due to liver vascularity.
c. The patient will be tired after the procedure and should get some rest.
d. Bed rest is maintained in order to prevent stitches from opening.

22. Which of the following is the antidote to warfarin (Coumadin)?

a. Magnesium sulfate
b. Protamine sulfate
c. Vitamin K
d. Saline

23. A female client who has just had gastrointestinal surgery states that she "Can't wait to go home and drink a soda." The nurse takes this to mean the patient has:

a. understood the discharge instructions. The patient can drink whatever she likes when she returns home.
b. misunderstood the discharge instructions. Carbonated beverages should be avoided for 3 to 4 weeks postoperatively.
c. misunderstood the discharge instructions. The patient should wait 24 hours before eating or drinking after discharge.
d. understood the discharge instructions and is repeating what the nurse told her.

24. For which of the following procedures would the McBurney incision be used?

a. Open appendectomy
b. Cesarean section
c. Spinal surgery
d. Oophorectomy

25. Sterile gowns are considered sterile:

a. from the neckline in front, from the shoulders to the level of the sterile field, and at the sleeves from 1 inch above the elbows including the cuffs.
b. in front from the shoulders to the level of the sterile field and at the sleeves from 2 inches above the elbows to the cuffs.
c. from the neckline in front and back, from the shoulders to the level of the sterile field, and at the sleeves from 1 inch above the elbows to the cuffs.
d. in front from the axillary area to the level of the sterile field and at the sleeves from 2 inches below the elbows to the cuffs.

26. The RNFA, acting as first assistant, is asked to also perform scrub nurse duties during a routine tonsillectomy. Per guidelines set forth from the Association of periOperative Registered Nurses (AORN), is this acceptable?

a. No. The RNFA may act as both first assistant and scrub nurse only for high-risk surgeries.
b. Yes. The RNFA may act as scrub nurse and first assistant intraoperatively.
c. No. The RNFA should not take on scrub nurse duties while acting as the first assistant.
d. Yes. The RNFA is required to perform both duties if necessary.

27. The anesthesiologist and perioperative nurse are giving the patient hand-off report to the PACU nurse when the anesthesiologist's pager goes off. He immediately heads for the nearest telephone and asks the perioperative nurse to finish the report. Is this appropriate?

a. The anesthesiologist is not present at the PACU hand-off report.
b. No, the anesthesiologist should remain with the patient until the PACU nurse accepts responsibility for the patient's care.
c. No, he should have responded to the page and returned to the PACU later to finish his report.
d. No, he should have asked the perioperative nurse to respond to the page while he completed his part of the report.

28. What is a function of calcium (CA++) in the body?

a. Controls cellular osmotic pressure
b. Influences bone growth
c. Regulates kidney function
d. Contributes to the acid-base balance

29. A patient is admitted to the hospital with respiratory failure. What is the normal range for pO2?

a. 30–45 mm Hg
b. 105–130 mm Hg
c. 80–100 mm Hg
d. 50–60 mm Hg

30. What type of incision is typically used for an open cholecystectomy?

a. Subcostal or Kocher
b. Lower midline
c. Thoracoabdominal
d. Transpleural approach

31. Which of the following is used as an inhalational anesthetic?

a. Propofol
b. Succinylcholine
c. Metaxalone
d. Nitrous oxide

32. Please choose the best definition for insufflation:

a. Expansion of a body cavity with CO2 gas
b. Closing a wound using a laser
c. Injecting large amounts of saline into a body cavity
d. Using CO2 gas to clear the surgeon's field of view during knee surgery

33. A patient has arrived at the OR for a resection to remove a carcinoid lung tumor. She is crying and shaking. What is the best way that the nurse can console the patient?

a. Offer to get her a sedative.
b. Remind her that she will be cured once she wakes up after surgery.
c. Tell her to say a prayer.
d. Assure her that the team will give her the best care possible.

34. Why is glycopyrrolate given preoperatively?

a. To sedate the patient
b. To suppress secretions during surgery
c. To aid in coagulation
d. To decrease heart rate

35. A patient is scheduled for a total knee replacement. Which of the following is indicated for this patient prior to surgery?

a. Stop NSAIDs at least two weeks prior to surgery.
b. Bed rest for one week prior to surgery
c. A CAT scan
d. Heparin injections

36. Which type of suture is used at the distal end of an appendiceal stump?

a. Simple suture
b. Purse-string suture
c. Continuous suture
d. Mattress suture

37. DeBakey forceps:

a. are heavy toothed forceps.
b. are used for delicate tissues.
c. are used for handling packing gauze and prosthetics.
d. All of the above

38. Per standard precautions, the modes of transmission of pathogens include all of the following EXCEPT:

a. contact.
b. vector-borne.
c. airborne.
d. environmental.

39. Why would a surgeon attempt to carry out an incision in the direction of Langer's lines?

a. To mitigate scarring
b. To promote healing
c. To cut in a straight line
d. A and B

40. During which procedure would cottonoids be used?

a. Craniotomy
b. Appendectomy
c. Rhinoplasty
d. Arthroscopy

41. Which is a good general rule to use when using a simple suture to close a wound?

a. The distance between each suture should be 1 mm.
b. The width of each stitch equals the distance between the sutures.
c. The width of each stitch should equal 1 mm.
d. The distance between each suture should be twice the length of each stitch.

42. Which of the following instruments are generally included in a major laparotomy set?

a. Army retractor
b. Yankauer suction tip
c. Backhaus towel clamp
d. All of the above

43. During which procedure would a nerve stimulator be used?

a. Cholecystectomy
b. Total knee replacement
c. Acoustic neuroma removal
d. Open reduction and fixation of a femur fracture

44. A patient presents for a follow-up appointment a week after a laparotomy with a bright green-blue discoloration on his dressing. What is a possible cause of the discoloration?

a. Zinc-saline wet dressing
b. Pseudomonas aeruginosa infection
c. Staphylococcus aureus infection
d. Colloidal silver ointment

45. Please choose the correct order of a midline abdominal closure.

a. Subcuticular, peritoneum, fascia, muscle, subcutaneous, skin
b. Peritoneum, muscle, subcutaneous, subcuticular, skin
c. Peritoneum, fascia, muscle, subcuticular, subcutaneous, skin
d. Peritoneum, fascia, muscle, subcutaneous, subcuticular, skin

46. The Bunnell technique suture is often used to repair:

a. Bone
b. Tendon
c. Eye
d. Vaginal tissue

47. Which of the following is NOT a responsibility of the RNFA during the perioperative experience?

a. In collaboration with the surgeon, examines the surgical wound for sponges, needles/sharps, and instruments prior to counts.
b. Conducts ongoing assessment of the patient's condition and relevant patient responses throughout the perioperative experience.
c. Verifies that instruments function properly.
d. Controls the patient's pain and level of consciousness intraoperatively.

48. Which product is often used to achieve hemostasis of the bone flap during cranial surgery?

a. Mesh
b. Horsley's wax
c. Gelfoam
d. Electrocautery

49. In what position is the patient placed for a left nephrectomy?

a. Left lateral position
b. Left lateral kidney position
c. Right lateral position
d. Prone

50. Where is the gastrocnemius muscle found?

a. Medial thigh
b. Lower back
c. Anterolateral leg
d. Posterior leg

Answer Key and Explanations

1. C: The lithotomy position is commonly used for procedures that require a perineal approach, as the patient is placed in a supine position with both legs in stirrups. This position provides the surgeon with good visual and physical access to the perineal area. It is used for gynecologic, rectal, and urologic procedures and is commonly used in the United States for childbirth. There are four levels of lithotomy: the low lithotomy, standard lithotomy, high lithotomy and exaggerated lithotomy.

2. D: Retractors are surgical instruments used to hold back wound edges, tissues, or other structures in order to provide exposure of the operative site. There are two types of retractors: self-retaining and hand-held or manual retractors. Self-retaining retractors have two or more opposing blades separated by a spring or ratchet. These types of retractors do not need to be held once inserted. Manual retractors have some sort of handle with a blade at a right angle. A malleable or ribbon retractor is a flat piece of metal that can be shaped at the field.

3. B: The spinal cord is surrounded by three meninges: the dura mater, the arachnoid mater, and the pia mater. The dura mater is the outermost layer and the most durable. It is separated from the spinal column by a layer of fat. Beneath the dura mater is the arachnoid mater, a thin membrane that is pressed against the inner surface of the dura mater. It is held in place by CSF pressure from the subarachnoid space, which is the space between the arachnoid mater and the pia mater. The pia mater is the innermost and most delicate of the meninges.

4. A: The left lung is divided into an upper and lower lobe separated by an oblique fissure. The right lung is divided into three lobes: the superior, middle, and inferior lobes. Each lung is composed of 10 major segments, with each segment having its own bronchus and branches of the pulmonary artery and vein. The apex of each lung projects above the first rib and the bases rest on the diaphragm. The main function of the lung is to exchange carbon dioxide for oxygen.

5. C: A Grade I surgical complication is defined as any deviation from the normal postoperative course that does not require pharmacological treatment or surgical, radiological, or endoscopic interventions. According to the Clavien-Dindo Classification of Surgical Complications, allowed therapeutic regimens for a Grade I complication include certain drugs such as antiemetics, antipyretics, diuretics, analgesics, and electrolytes, as well as physiotherapy. This grade also includes wound infections that are opened at the bedside. Examples of Grade I complications include noninfectious diarrhea and a transient elevation of serum creatinine.

6. C: The Brush-Stroke method is an aseptic technique used during surgical scrub and includes, for each arm and hand, scrubbing nails 30 strokes; each side of each finger, starting with the thumb, 20 strokes; the back of the hand 20 strokes; the palm of the hand 20 strokes; the arm 20 strokes for each 1/3 and each side, to 2 inches above the elbow. Prior to scrubbing in, all jewelry should be removed from the hands and forearms. Fingernails should be short, clean, and healthy. The healthcare professional should also be free of open wounds, abrasions, weeping rashes, or fresh tattoos on exposed skin areas.

7. C: Obese surgical patients are more susceptible to compromised skin integrity, including shearing. Decreased oxygen tension at the tissue level in patients with obesity places the patient at greater risk for infection and tissue hypoxia. They are also more likely to develop deep vein thrombosis and pulmonary embolism, experience compromised ventilation, postoperative back pain, and pressure ulcers. Proper patient positioning, including head, shoulder, and upper body elevation to facilitate airway alignment, and suitable equipment are essential for this population.

8. A: Midazolam (Versed) is often given to alleviate apprehension, induce sedation, and provide amnesia during procedures. For most patients, it has a short duration and fast recovery time. Patients given midazolam should be monitored closely for hypotension, due to a reduction in systemic vascular resistance. Other common side effects of Versed include confusion, amnesia, weakness, chills, apnea, nausea and vomiting, and respiratory depression. Apnea, respiratory depression, and amnesia may be more pronounced in the elderly.

9. A: During the proliferative phase of wound healing, granulation occurs when fibroblasts create a collagen bed to fill the wound and grow a new network of blood vessels. A new epithelium provides a protective covering that reduces the risk of infection and provides a barrier to fluid loss. As the wound is undergoing re-epithelialization, wound contraction occurs, thus shrinking the area of the wound.

10. C: Collagen sutures are absorbable and will break down in the body over time. These sutures are utilized internally so wound reopening is not required. Collagen sutures are also commonly used for the eyes. Other types of absorbable sutures include surgical gut and synthetic absorbable sutures, made from a combination of lactic acid and glycolic acid polymers. Non-absorbable sutures will not break down in tissue and include cotton, silk, nylon, polyester, and stainless steel.

11. D: A clean-contaminated wound should have no signs of infection. These operative wounds occur when the respiratory, genitourinary, or alimentary tracts are entered under controlled conditions. A gunshot wound is an example of a contaminated wound, a perforated viscera is an example of a dirty wound, and a breast biopsy is an example of a clean wound.

12. D: An infant's body water content is approximately 70% to 80%. Infants and very young children are at a higher risk of fluid imbalance because a greater percentage of their body weight is in water. This greater percentage of fluid contributes to a decreased ability to compensate for fluid loss. Adults are generally 60% water, while the elderly usually are 45% to 55% body water.

13. B: The nurse is using the closed-gloving technique. The gloves are handled through the fabric of the gown sleeves and the hands are not extended from the sleeves because the cuffs are considered unsterile. The glove cuff is stretched over the opening of the sleeve to cover the entire gown cuff. As the cuff is being drawn back, the nurse extends her hand and fingers into the glove. The closed gloving technique can only be used for initial gloving.

14. C: Vomiting is not generally associated with malignant hyperthermia. Malignant hyperthermia is a life-threatening complication that may be induced by drugs used for anesthesia. Succinylcholine and inhalation anesthetics are often considered causal agents. Other common signs of malignant hyperthermia include tachypnea, muscle rigidity, metabolic and respiratory acidosis, unstable blood pressure, and rising body temperature.

15. A: Placing a pillow under the patient's lower legs will suspend the heels off the operating room bed, thus diminishing pressure on that area. The heel is very sensitive to developing pressure-related ulcers, even when placed on pressure-reducing beds and other devices. Other pressure-reducing measures include using pressure-relieving mattresses, padding around firm or rigid surfaces, and performing passive range of motion exercises to limbs every 1–2 hours.

16. A: Immediately following exposure to blood-borne pathogens from a needle stick or other sharps injury, the injured party should rinse the area with water and clean the wound with soap or a disinfectant. The nurse manager should be alerted, the source patient should be identified, and the injured person should go to employee health or the emergency department. In most cases, a post-exposure treatment plan is put into place.

17. B: Sterile defogging solutions can be applied to the endoscopic lens in order to create a coating and reduce fogging. Lens fogging occurs when the cool metal of the endoscope comes in contact with the warmth of the body. Warming the endoscope with sponges soaked in warm sterile water or using sterile scope warmers are other options that can help prevent lens fogging, thus reducing frustration and saving time.

18. B: Wound debridement is performed in order to remove dead or devitalized tissue from a wound. This is important in order to prevent infection caused by the dead tissue. There are several debridement options including surgical wound debridement, biologic debridement (i.e., sterile maggot therapy), mechanical debridement (i.e., wet-to-dry dressings), chemical or enzymatic debridement (i.e., using a pharmaceutical version of collagenase), or autolytic debridement (i.e., using dressings to help the body use its own abilities to dissolve the dead tissue).

19. C: Ischemic optic neuropathy (ION) is the most common cause of perioperative visual loss. Increased intraocular pressure can occur when there is indirect or direct pressure on the globe of the eye. The prone position increases intraocular pressure, especially when prone Trendelenburg's position is used. Prolonged procedures, which can contribute to decreased perfusion to the optic nerve and excessive blood loss, are additional risk factors, as are patient co-morbidities of diabetes, hypertension, and anemia. Prevention is key as there is no current established treatment for ION.

20. B: A continuous suture is made with one uninterrupted length of suture. Only the first and last stitches are tied. A continuous suture would be used to close tissue that needs a tight closure, such as on blood vessels to prevent leakage. Other types of sutures include an interrupted suture in which each stitch is tied individually, a stay or retention suture which is used to reinforce the primary suture, subcuticular sutures in which the stitch is placed under the epidermal skin layer, and the purse-string suture which surrounds a circular wound opening.

21. B: Due to liver vascularity there is a high risk of bleeding or hemorrhage following a liver biopsy. Bed rest can help prevent injury and promote healing. The patient should lie on the right side for a minimum of two hours following the biopsy and maintain bed rest for up to 12 hours. Recovery is expected within one to two days; however, pain at the incision site may persist for several days and should be managed with prescribed pain medication.

22. C: Vitamin K is the antidote to warfarin. Warfarin is an anticoagulant that inhibits the effects of vitamin K on clotting factor II, factor XII, factor IX, and factor X. Warfarin blocks the action of vitamin K within the liver by competing for the same absorption sites needed for vitamin K uptake. Therefore, the levels of vitamin K within the liver decrease. Patients taking warfarin should be advised to limit their intake of foods high in vitamin K such as leafy greens, Brussels sprouts, and broccoli. Protamine sulfate is the antidote for heparin.

23. B: Patients should avoid carbonated beverages for 3 to 4 weeks after GI surgery to help prevent gas and bloating. The nurse could take this opportunity to re-educate the patient on the discharge instructions. Other general discharge instructions for a patient who has undergone GI surgery include adding solid foods back into the diet gradually, eating small but frequent meals, keeping the wound area clean and dry, and checking the incisional area daily for redness, swelling, and discharge.

24. A: The McBurney incision is commonly used for an open appendectomy. McBurney's point is located about two thirds of the distance from the anterior superior iliac spine in the right lower quadrant to the umbilicus. It is an oblique incision in which the external oblique muscle and fascia are split and retracted. The internal oblique muscle, transverse muscle, and fascia are also split and retracted. It is a quick incision that is easy to close.

25. B: Sterile gowns are considered sterile in front from the shoulders to the level of the sterile field and at the sleeves from two inches above the elbows to the cuffs. The cuffs, neckline, axillary area, shoulders, and the back of the gown are considered unsterile. Cuffs are not an effective barrier to bacteria and should be covered by sterile gloves.

26. C: According to the Association of periOperative Registered Nurses (AORN), intraoperatively, the registered nurse first assistant (RNFA) acts under the direction of the surgeon and should not function concurrently as the scrub nurse. The role of the RNFA is to work with the surgeon and the surgical team using instruments and medical devices, cutting and suturing tissue, providing hemostasis and exposure to the surgical field, and other intraoperative surgical assistant tasks.

27. B: Per guidelines from The Joint Commission, interruptions during the hand-off report should be kept to a minimum. The members of the surgical team should not answer pages or cause interruption during the hand-off. Neither the anesthesiologist nor perioperative nurse should leave the patient in the PACU until the PACU nurse accepts the responsibility for the nursing care of the patient. It is important that the PACU nurse is given the opportunity to review the reports and has time to answer any questions he/she may have regarding the care of the patient.

28. B: Calcium (Ca++) helps to influence bone building and growth. It also helps regulate blood pressure, contributes to brain function, and is used in blood clotting. Among other functions, potassium (K+) helps control cellular osmotic pressure, sodium (NA+) influences the kidney's regulation of water and electrolyte status, and chlorides (Cl-) contribute to the acid-base balance.

29. C: The normal range for p02 is 80–100 mm Hg. P02 (or partial pressure of oxygen) reflects the amount of dissolved oxygen in the blood. It measures the effectiveness of the lungs in pulling oxygen into the bloodstream from the atmosphere. It is measured in mm Hg (millimeters of mercury). Increased levels may indicate excessive oxygen intake, and decreased levels may indicate COPD, asthma, and other causes of hypoxia.

30. A: For an open cholecystectomy the abdominal cavity is opened through a right subcostal or Kocher incision. An upper midline incision can also be used; however, these are painful and restrict pulmonary function. The subcostal incision affords greater lateral exposure for the surgeon and less pain for the surgical patient. The subcostal incision does generally cause the operation to take longer as there are more layers to suture.

31. D: Nitrous oxide can be used as an inhalational anesthetic agent. After inhalation, it is absorbed by diffusion through the lungs and eliminated by normal respiration. It is often used with oxygen in combination with more potent gases for surgical anesthesia in pediatric patients. Nitrous oxide is also commonly used for dental procedures. Succinylcholine and propofol are administered intravenously. Metaxalone is an oral muscle relaxant.

32. A: Expansion of a body cavity with carbon dioxide gas (C02) can be defined as insufflation. This is used in the abdomen for laparoscopic procedures so that space is created for the endoscopic camera to view the cavity and for the surgeon to work. A 1 mm incision is made below the umbilicus and the Veress needle is passed through the incision. Once it is in the proper position, the needle is connected to the insufflator and the CO_2 gas is infused into the cavity. This is done first at low pressure to ensure the needle is in the proper position. Once that is established, flow rate can be increased. 12–15 mm Hg is the usual pressure for a laparoscopy.

33. D: The best way the nurse can console the patient would be to assure her that the surgical team would provide her with the best care possible. It would not be appropriate to offer her a sedative, as that could interfere with the anesthesiologist's plan of care and not address the immediate psychosocial needs of the patient. There is no guarantee that the surgery will cure the patient, therefore it is misleading to placate the patient by advising her she will be cured post-surgery. Though it may be comforting for the patient to pray, this should not be suggested unless the patient has expressed interest in prayer. The nurse needs to be sensitive to the beliefs and religious choices of the patient.

34. B: Glycopyrrolate (Robinul) is an anticholinergic that is given preoperatively to suppress oral, gastric, and respiratory secretions during surgery. Glycopyrrolate also increases heart rate in order to prevent bradycardia. Other anticholinergic agents that may be given preoperatively include atropine and scopolamine eye drops (for eye surgeries).

35. A: Though some physicians opt to stop NSAIDs earlier, in general, NSAIDs should be stopped at least three days prior to surgery. NSAIDs such as naproxen or ibuprofen diminish platelet aggregation and can increase bleeding time and overall bleeding risk. Since NSAIDs can be obtained over-the-counter, it is very important to receive an accurate medication history from the patient prior to the procedure.

36. B: A purse-string suture of 3-0 absorbable suture should be placed around the appendiceal stump. A purse-string suture is a running stitch suture that is placed around the edge of a circular wound so that when the ends of the suture are drawn together its appearance is that of a drawstring purse. During an appendectomy, a Kelly clamp is used to invert the stump of the appendix as the purse-string suture is tied. This creates an inverted stump.

37. B: DeBakey forceps are generally used to grasp delicate tissues without trauma. They are often used in abdominal and vascular surgeries and are suitable for handling bowel, blood vessels, and bile ducts. They are also commonly used in cardiovascular surgeries. DeBakey forceps usually require a specific spring tension in order to open and close without unnecessary force that could damage sensitive tissues.

38. D: Modes of transmission for disease include airborne (including droplet transmission), vector-borne, contact, and common vehicle. Airborne transmission occurs when droplet particles travel at least three feet through the air and come in contact with the mucous membranes. This can happen during talking, sneezing, or suctioning. Vector-borne transmission occurs from one host to another via an animal transfer, such as a mosquito. Contact transmission occurs either directly, from person to person, or indirectly, from person to inanimate object to person.

Common vehicle transmission takes place when pathogens are spread through a common reservoir such as food or water.

39. D: Langer's lines run parallel to the predominant direction of collagen bundles in the dermis. Karl Langer first described them in 1861, after he punched holes in a cadaver and noted that the punctures in the skin created ellipsoidal shapes that produced line directions. Therefore, incisions made parallel to Langer's lines generally heal better and produce less scarring than incisions made perpendicular to the lines. This is especially important in plastic surgery.

40. A: Cottonoids are used for hemostasis and delicate tissue protection. For example, cottonoid patties are used in neurosurgery to protect the delicate membranes of the brain. It is less traumatic if suctioning is performed over a patty rather than directly on the tissue. They are also often used in laminectomies. Patties are made of cotton or rayon and come in strips or squares. There is a string and sensor attached to the patty that will show up on an x-ray.

41. B: A good general rule for the placement of stitches when using a simple suture is that the width of each stitch equals the distance between the sutures. The width of the stitch will vary with the purpose of the suture and the location of the wound, as well as the thickness of the skin. The simple suture should also have a square-shaped profile in order to avoid inverting the edges of the skin.

42. D: Though general surgical instrumentation will vary per hospital or surgeon preference, some of the parts of a major laparotomy set are as follows: Army retractor, Yankauer suction tip, Backhaus towel clamp, DeBakey forceps, straight and curved Mayo scissors, Russian tissue forceps, Cushing tissue forceps, ribbon retractor, Kelly retractor, and several sizes of Mayo-Hegar needle holders.

43. C: A nerve stimulator is useful during acoustic neuroma removal to identify the seventh cranial nerve. As this nerve controls several facial movements, it is important to know the exact location of this nerve during surgery in order to avoid damage that could result in facial palsy or paralysis. During operation of a nerve stimulator, the needle that is attached to a probe is passed through the adjacent tissue. A very small electric current is delivered through the probe to the structure in question. Once stimulated, the nerve will move.

44. B: The most likely cause of the blue-green discoloration on the dressing is a Pseudomonas aeruginosa colonization. Pseudomonas aeruginosa is a gram-negative bacteria that secretes several pigments including pyocyanin, which can be identified by its blue-green color. It also produces a pungent odor that can be described as fruity or like sweat socks. It thrives on most surfaces and can be found on medical equipment, causing cross-contamination.

45. D: The correct order of closure for a midline abdominal incision from inner to outer layer is: peritoneum, fascia, muscle, subcutaneous, subcuticular, and finally, skin. There are differing ideologies and techniques when performing a closure on a midline abdominal incision. For example, some surgeons choose not to close the peritoneum; there is not sufficient scientific evidence to show that this is necessary. Closure of the fascia is also variable among surgeons. The two primary methods are layered closure, where each layer is closed individually, and mass closure, which is continuous fascial closure with a single suture.

46. B: The Bunnell technique suture, also called a "pull-out suture," is often used in tendon repair. The suture is placed through the incision in order to be pulled out once its function to hold the tendon together is no longer needed. After approximating the tendon ends, the two ends of the suture are brought out through the skin and tied together over a button. If using a modified Bunnell stitch, a square knot is made with the free ends of the suture and remains buried within the tendon. These types of sutures are often used for tendon repair in the hands and fingers.

47. D: Though the RNFA is responsible for conducting an ongoing assessment of the patient's condition and relevant patient responses throughout the perioperative experience, it is the anesthesiologist's duty to control the patient's pain and level of consciousness intraoperatively. Per the Association of periOperative Registered Nurses (AORN), the RNFA is responsible for the four domains of nursing activities included in the competency statements taken from the Perioperative Nursing Data Set. The domains are as follows: Safety, Physiologic Responses, Behavioral – Patient and Family: Knowledge and Rights/Ethics, and Health System.

48. B: Horsley's wax, or bone wax, is very effective in controlling bleeding from the bone flap created during neurosurgery. Considerable bleeding can occur due to the highly vascular red bone marrow found inside this structure. The surgeon lessens the bleeding by spreading the wax over the cut surfaces of the bone. Sir Victor Haden Horsley created the wax in 1892 from beeswax, though different components have been added since its creation. Large amounts of bone wax should be avoided as the body may identify the wax as a foreign body and a source of infection, requiring a secondary removal.

49. C: The patient should be positioned in the right lateral position for a left open nephrectomy with the dependent iliac crest placed over the kidney rest. This position is a modification of the jackknife position. A pillow should be placed between the legs, with the lower leg bent at the knee and the upper leg extended. Adhesive tape or a strap is used across the hips for stabilizing the body. The upper arm is supported on an overhead arm support and the lower arm on a padded armboard.

50. D: The gastrocnemius muscle is part of the calf muscle and is found on the posterior, or back part, of the lower leg. This muscle is responsible for plantar flexion of the ankle and non-weight bearing knee flexion, and also stabilizes the ankle and knee when standing. It is used in walking, running, and jumping. Common injuries include strains and tears.

How to Overcome Test Anxiety

Just the thought of taking a test is enough to make most people a little nervous. A test is an important event that can have a long-term impact on your future, so it's important to take it seriously and it's natural to feel anxious about performing well. But just because anxiety is normal, that doesn't mean that it's helpful in test taking, or that you should simply accept it as part of your life. Anxiety can have a variety of effects. These effects can be mild, like making you feel slightly nervous, or severe, like blocking your ability to focus or remember even a simple detail.

If you experience test anxiety—whether severe or mild—it's important to know how to beat it. To discover this, first you need to understand what causes test anxiety.

Causes of Test Anxiety

While we often think of anxiety as an uncontrollable emotional state, it can actually be caused by simple, practical things. One of the most common causes of test anxiety is that a person does not feel adequately prepared for their test. This feeling can be the result of many different issues such as poor study habits or lack of organization, but the most common culprit is time management. Starting to study too late, failing to organize your study time to cover all of the material, or being distracted while you study will mean that you're not well prepared for the test. This may lead to cramming the night before, which will cause you to be physically and mentally exhausted for the test. Poor time management also contributes to feelings of stress, fear, and hopelessness as you realize you are not well prepared but don't know what to do about it.

Other times, test anxiety is not related to your preparation for the test but comes from unresolved fear. This may be a past failure on a test, or poor performance on tests in general. It may come from comparing yourself to others who seem to be performing better or from the stress of living up to expectations. Anxiety may be driven by fears of the future—how failure on this test would affect your educational and career goals. These fears are often completely irrational, but they can still negatively impact your test performance.

Elements of Test Anxiety

As mentioned earlier, test anxiety is considered to be an emotional state, but it has physical and mental components as well. Sometimes you may not even realize that you are suffering from test anxiety until you notice the physical symptoms. These can include trembling hands, rapid heartbeat, sweating, nausea, and tense muscles. Extreme anxiety may lead to fainting or vomiting. Obviously, any of these symptoms can have a negative impact on testing. It is important to recognize them as soon as they begin to occur so that you can address the problem before it damages your performance.

The mental components of test anxiety include trouble focusing and inability to remember learned information. During a test, your mind is on high alert, which can help you recall information and stay focused for an extended period of time. However, anxiety interferes with your mind's natural processes, causing you to blank out, even on the questions you know well. The strain of testing during anxiety makes it difficult to stay focused, especially on a test that may take several hours. Extreme anxiety can take a huge mental toll, making it difficult not only to recall test information but even to understand the test questions or pull your thoughts together.

Effects of Test Anxiety

Test anxiety is like a disease—if left untreated, it will get progressively worse. Anxiety leads to poor performance, and this reinforces the feelings of fear and failure, which in turn lead to poor performances on subsequent tests. It can grow from a mild nervousness to a crippling condition. If allowed to progress, test anxiety can have a big impact on your schooling, and consequently on your future.

Test anxiety can spread to other parts of your life. Anxiety on tests can become anxiety in any stressful situation, and blanking on a test can turn into panicking in a job situation. But fortunately, you don't have to let anxiety rule your testing and determine your grades. There are a number of relatively simple steps you can take to move past anxiety and function normally on a test and in the rest of life.

Physical Steps for Beating Test Anxiety

While test anxiety is a serious problem, the good news is that it can be overcome. It doesn't have to control your ability to think and remember information. While it may take time, you can begin taking steps today to beat anxiety.

Just as your first hint that you may be struggling with anxiety comes from the physical symptoms, the first step to treating it is also physical. Rest is crucial for having a clear, strong mind. If you are tired, it is much easier to give in to anxiety. But if you establish good sleep habits, your body and mind will be ready to perform optimally, without the strain of exhaustion. Additionally, sleeping well helps you to retain information better, so you're more likely to recall the answers when you see the test questions.

Getting good sleep means more than going to bed on time. It's important to allow your brain time to relax. Take study breaks from time to time so it doesn't get overworked, and don't study right before bed. Take time to rest your mind before trying to rest your body, or you may find it difficult to fall asleep.

Along with sleep, other aspects of physical health are important in preparing for a test. Good nutrition is vital for good brain function. Sugary foods and drinks may give a burst of energy but this burst is followed by a crash, both physically and emotionally. Instead, fuel your body with protein and vitamin-rich foods.

Also, drink plenty of water. Dehydration can lead to headaches and exhaustion, especially if your brain is already under stress from the rigors of the test. Particularly if your test is a long one, drink water during the breaks. And if possible, take an energy-boosting snack to eat between sections.

Along with sleep and diet, a third important part of physical health is exercise. Maintaining a steady workout schedule is helpful, but even taking 5-minute study breaks to walk can help get your blood pumping faster and clear your head. Exercise also releases endorphins, which contribute to a positive feeling and can help combat test anxiety.

When you nurture your physical health, you are also contributing to your mental health. If your body is healthy, your mind is much more likely to be healthy as well. So take time to rest, nourish your body with healthy food and water, and get moving as much as possible. Taking these physical steps will make you stronger and more able to take the mental steps necessary to overcome test anxiety.

Mental Steps for Beating Test Anxiety

Working on the mental side of test anxiety can be more challenging, but as with the physical side, there are clear steps you can take to overcome it. As mentioned earlier, test anxiety often stems from lack of preparation, so the obvious solution is to prepare for the test. Effective studying may be the most important weapon you have for beating test anxiety, but you can and should employ several other mental tools to combat fear.

First, boost your confidence by reminding yourself of past success—tests or projects that you aced. If you're putting as much effort into preparing for this test as you did for those, there's no reason you should expect to fail here. Work hard to prepare; then trust your preparation.

Second, surround yourself with encouraging people. It can be helpful to find a study group, but be sure that the people you're around will encourage a positive attitude. If you spend time with others who are anxious or cynical, this will only contribute to your own anxiety. Look for others who are motivated to study hard from a desire to succeed, not from a fear of failure.

Third, reward yourself. A test is physically and mentally tiring, even without anxiety, and it can be helpful to have something to look forward to. Plan an activity following the test, regardless of the outcome, such as going to a movie or getting ice cream.

When you are taking the test, if you find yourself beginning to feel anxious, remind yourself that you know the material. Visualize successfully completing the test. Then take a few deep, relaxing breaths and return to it. Work through the questions carefully but with confidence, knowing that you are capable of succeeding.

Developing a healthy mental approach to test taking will also aid in other areas of life. Test anxiety affects more than just the actual test—it can be damaging to your mental health and even contribute to depression. It's important to beat test anxiety before it becomes a problem for more than testing.

Study Strategy

Being prepared for the test is necessary to combat anxiety, but what does being prepared look like? You may study for hours on end and still not feel prepared. What you need is a strategy for test prep. The next few pages outline our recommended steps to help you plan out and conquer the challenge of preparation.

Step 1: Scope Out the Test

Learn everything you can about the format (multiple choice, essay, etc.) and what will be on the test. Gather any study materials, course outlines, or sample exams that may be available. Not only will this help you to prepare, but knowing what to expect can help to alleviate test anxiety.

Step 2: Map Out the Material

Look through the textbook or study guide and make note of how many chapters or sections it has. Then divide these over the time you have. For example, if a book has 15 chapters and you have five days to study, you need to cover three chapters each day. Even better, if you have the time, leave an extra day at the end for overall review after you have gone through the material in depth.

If time is limited, you may need to prioritize the material. Look through it and make note of which sections you think you already have a good grasp on, and which need review. While you are studying, skim quickly through the familiar sections and take more time on the challenging parts. Write out your plan so you don't get lost as you go. Having a written plan also helps you feel more in control of the study, so anxiety is less likely to arise from feeling overwhelmed at the amount to cover.

Step 3: Gather Your Tools

Decide what study method works best for you. Do you prefer to highlight in the book as you study and then go back over the highlighted portions? Or do you type out notes of the important information? Or is it helpful to make flashcards that you can carry with you? Assemble the pens, index cards, highlighters, post-it notes, and any other materials you may need so you won't be distracted by getting up to find things while you study.

If you're having a hard time retaining the information or organizing your notes, experiment with different methods. For example, try color-coding by subject with colored pens, highlighters, or post-it notes. If you learn better by hearing, try recording yourself reading your notes so you can listen while in the car, working out, or simply sitting at your desk. Ask a friend to quiz you from your flashcards, or try teaching someone the material to solidify it in your mind.

Step 4: Create Your Environment

It's important to avoid distractions while you study. This includes both the obvious distractions like visitors and the subtle distractions like an uncomfortable chair (or a too-comfortable couch that makes you want to fall asleep). Set up the best study environment possible: good lighting and a comfortable work area. If background music helps you focus, you may want to turn it on, but otherwise keep the room quiet. If you are using a computer to take notes, be sure you don't have any other windows open, especially applications like social media, games, or anything else that could distract you. Silence your phone and turn off notifications. Be sure to keep water close by so you stay hydrated while you study (but avoid unhealthy drinks and snacks).

Also, take into account the best time of day to study. Are you freshest first thing in the morning? Try to set aside some time then to work through the material. Is your mind clearer in the afternoon or evening? Schedule your study session then. Another method is to study at the same time of day that you will take the test, so that your brain gets used to working on the material at that time and will be ready to focus at test time.

Step 5: Study!

Once you have done all the study preparation, it's time to settle into the actual studying. Sit down, take a few moments to settle your mind so you can focus, and begin to follow your study plan. Don't give in to distractions or let yourself procrastinate. This is your time to prepare so you'll be ready to fearlessly approach the test. Make the most of the time and stay focused.

Of course, you don't want to burn out. If you study too long you may find that you're not retaining the information very well. Take regular study breaks. For example, taking five minutes out of every hour to walk briskly, breathing deeply and swinging your arms, can help your mind stay fresh.

As you get to the end of each chapter or section, it's a good idea to do a quick review. Remind yourself of what you learned and work on any difficult parts. When you feel that you've mastered the material, move on to the next part. At the end of your study session, briefly skim through your notes again.

But while review is helpful, cramming last minute is NOT. If at all possible, work ahead so that you won't need to fit all your study into the last day. Cramming overloads your brain with more information than it can process and retain, and your tired mind may struggle to recall even previously learned information when it is overwhelmed with last-minute study. Also, the urgent nature of cramming and the stress placed on your brain contribute to anxiety. You'll be more likely to go to the test feeling unprepared and having trouble thinking clearly.

So don't cram, and don't stay up late before the test, even just to review your notes at a leisurely pace. Your brain needs rest more than it needs to go over the information again. In fact, plan to finish your studies by noon or early afternoon the day before the test. Give your brain the rest of the day to relax or focus on other things, and get a good night's sleep. Then you will be fresh for the test and better able to recall what you've studied.

STEP 6: TAKE A PRACTICE TEST

Many courses offer sample tests, either online or in the study materials. This is an excellent resource to check whether you have mastered the material, as well as to prepare for the test format and environment.

Check the test format ahead of time: the number of questions, the type (multiple choice, free response, etc.), and the time limit. Then create a plan for working through them. For example, if you have 30 minutes to take a 60-question test, your limit is 30 seconds per question. Spend less time on the questions you know well so that you can take more time on the difficult ones.

If you have time to take several practice tests, take the first one open book, with no time limit. Work through the questions at your own pace and make sure you fully understand them. Gradually work up to taking a test under test conditions: sit at a desk with all study materials put away and set a timer. Pace yourself to make sure you finish the test with time to spare and go back to check your answers if you have time.

After each test, check your answers. On the questions you missed, be sure you understand why you missed them. Did you misread the question (tests can use tricky wording)? Did you forget the information? Or was it something you hadn't learned? Go back and study any shaky areas that the practice tests reveal.

Taking these tests not only helps with your grade, but also aids in combating test anxiety. If you're already used to the test conditions, you're less likely to worry about it, and working through tests until you're scoring well gives you a confidence boost. Go through the practice tests until you feel comfortable, and then you can go into the test knowing that you're ready for it.

Test Tips

On test day, you should be confident, knowing that you've prepared well and are ready to answer the questions. But aside from preparation, there are several test day strategies you can employ to maximize your performance.

First, as stated before, get a good night's sleep the night before the test (and for several nights before that, if possible). Go into the test with a fresh, alert mind rather than staying up late to study.

Try not to change too much about your normal routine on the day of the test. It's important to eat a nutritious breakfast, but if you normally don't eat breakfast at all, consider eating just a protein bar. If you're a coffee drinker, go ahead and have your normal coffee. Just make sure you time it so that the caffeine doesn't wear off right in the middle of your test. Avoid sugary beverages, and drink enough water to stay hydrated but not so much that you need a restroom break 10 minutes into the test. If your test isn't first thing in the morning, consider going for a walk or doing a light workout before the test to get your blood flowing.

Allow yourself enough time to get ready, and leave for the test with plenty of time to spare so you won't have the anxiety of scrambling to arrive in time. Another reason to be early is to select a good seat. It's helpful to sit away from doors and windows, which can be distracting. Find a good seat, get out your supplies, and settle your mind before the test begins.

When the test begins, start by going over the instructions carefully, even if you already know what to expect. Make sure you avoid any careless mistakes by following the directions.

Then begin working through the questions, pacing yourself as you've practiced. If you're not sure on an answer, don't spend too much time on it, and don't let it shake your confidence. Either skip it and come back later, or eliminate as many wrong answers as possible and guess among the remaining ones. Don't dwell on these questions as you continue—put them out of your mind and focus on what lies ahead.

Be sure to read all of the answer choices, even if you're sure the first one is the right answer. Sometimes you'll find a better one if you keep reading. But don't second-guess yourself if you do immediately know the answer. Your gut instinct is usually right. Don't let test anxiety rob you of the information you know.

If you have time at the end of the test (and if the test format allows), go back and review your answers. Be cautious about changing any, since your first instinct tends to be correct, but make sure you didn't misread any of the questions or accidentally mark the wrong answer choice. Look over any you skipped and make an educated guess.

At the end, leave the test feeling confident. You've done your best, so don't waste time worrying about your performance or wishing you could change anything. Instead, celebrate the successful completion of this test. And finally, use this test to learn how to deal with anxiety even better next time.

Review Video: Test Anxiety
Visit mometrix.com/academy and enter code: 100340

Important Qualification

Not all anxiety is created equal. If your test anxiety is causing major issues in your life beyond the classroom or testing center, or if you are experiencing troubling physical symptoms related to your anxiety, it may be a sign of a serious physiological or psychological condition. If this sounds like your situation, we strongly encourage you to seek professional help.

Online Resources

Due to our efforts to try to keep this book to a manageable length, we've created a link that will give you access to all of your online resources:

mometrix.com/resources719/crnfa

It's Your Moment, Let's Celebrate It!

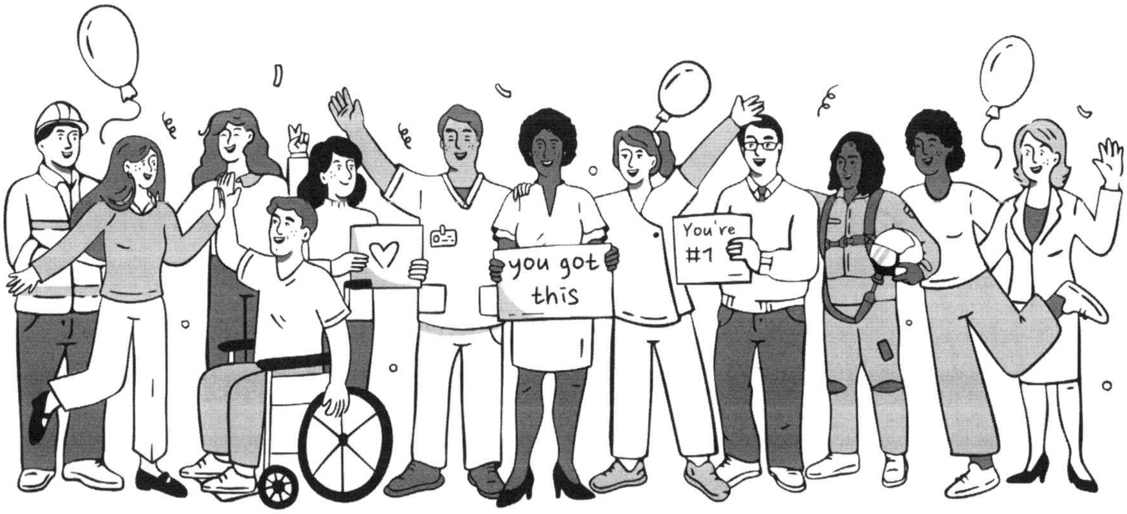

Share your story @mometrixtestpreparation